It's OK to have L̲_̲_̲_̲ in Your Lipstick

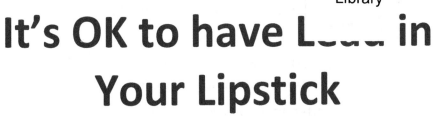

and answers to other beauty questions that you're dying to know

Written by Perry Romanowski & Randy Schueller

Edited by Lily Elderkin

Published in the United States by Brains Publishing.
www.brainspublishing.com

The authors have attempted to make this book as accurate and up to date as possible, but it may contain errors, omissions, or material that is out of date at the time you read it. Neither the author nor publisher has any legal responsibility or liability for errors, omissions, out-of-date material, or the reader's application of the advice contained in this book

First edition

ISBN 10: 0-9802173-6-9

ISBN 13: 978-0-9802173-6-0

Book design: Y42K Book Production Services

http://www.y42k.com/bookproduction.html

What others are saying about
the Beauty Brains new book

"The Beauty Brains are a group of scientists after my own heart: They do a great job of cutting through misleading info to explain which cosmetic ingredients are bad for your skin, which are brilliant, and when what you've heard or read is simply scare tactics."

—Paula Begoun, best-selling author of "Don't Go to the Cosmetics Counter Without Me"

"As a beauty editor, I'm bombarded with dozens of marketing claims and hyberbolic product testimonials on a daily basis by various beauty companies. I really appreciate the dose of science-based common sense the Beauty Brains dish out. It helps me write about beauty products and introduce them to readers in a more truthful, balanced way."

—Cheryl Wischhover, Beauty Editor, Fashionista.com (http://fashionista.com/)

"This is the best beauty bible I've ever read. Never get duped again after reading the most up-to-date information on the latest skin, hair and makeup products."

—Lora Condon aka The Beauty Buster Author of "Spa Wars—The Ugly Truth About the Beauty Industry"

"Every day we are bombarded with hype, fear-mongering, and ridiculous claims about our beauty products. Will this cream really erase my wrinkles? Will that lotion cause cancer? In "It's OK to have Lead in your Lipstick," the author of the web's premiere scientific resource on beauty products, The Beauty Brains, reveals the truth that cosmetics companies and health reporters haven't revealed. It's fun, fascinating, and a must-read for anyone who puts anything on their face! After reading this book, I'll rethink some of the recommendations I give to my patients!"

—Dr. Anthony Youn, M.D., F.A.C.S. Cosmetic surgeon blogger at Celebrity Cosmetic Surgery, and author of "In Stitches"

Acknowledgements

Perry and Randy would like to thank ALL the members of the Beauty Brains community without whom this book would not be possible. (Especially the more prolific members of our Forum who help answer questions while asking a few of their own!) Thanks guys!

Table of Contents

ACKNOWLEDGEMENTS 5

TABLE OF CONTENTS 6

INTRODUCTION 1

PART 1: CLEVER LIES THE BEAUTY COMPANIES TELL YOU 3

GENERAL QUESTIONS 4

SKIN CARE/MAKEUP QUESTIONS 29

HAIR CARE QUESTIONS 61

PART 2: SCAREMONGERING VERSUS TRULY SCARY (ARE COSMETICS SAFE?) 76

GENERAL QUESTIONS 77

SKIN CARE/MAKEUP QUESTIONS 107

HAIR CARE QUESTIONS 134

PART 3: MAKEUP OR MAKE BELIEVE (POPULAR BEAUTY MYTHS) 141

SKIN CARE/MAKEUP QUESTIONS 142

HAIR CARE QUESTIONS 176

PART 4: GREEN PRODUCTS - GREEN OR JUST GREENWASHED? ... 197

GENERAL QUESTIONS 198

SKIN CARE/MAKEUP QUESTIONS 213

HAIR CARE QUESTIONS 233

PART 5: BIZARRE BEAUTY INGREDIENTS 250

SKIN CARE/MAKEUP QUESTIONS 251

HAIR CARE QUESTIONS 283

PART 6: DOES ANYTHING REALLY WORK? 289

SKIN CARE/MAKEUP QUESTIONS 290

HAIR CARE QUESTIONS 325

APPENDIX **339**

WHERE TO LEARN MORE ABOUT BEAUTY SCIENCE 339

Introduction

Why should I read this book?

Read this book if you want to be a smarter shopper.

Smarter because you'll be able to spot over-hyped, over-priced beauty products. Smarter because you'll be able to shop for products you LOVE without worrying about which ingredient scare-story you should believe. Smarter because you'll be able to look your friends and family in the eyes and tell them "No, mineral oil in cosmetics does not cause cancer."

This book will change the way you think about beauty products

Being a smarter shopper, however, comes with a price. You like, many fans of our website, may find yourself turning into a "Beauty Brainiac." Symptoms of being a "Beauty Brainiac" include:

• Catching yourself reading the back of your shampoo bottle in the shower.

• Finding out who makes your favorite product and then checking to see if they make any other brands that have similar formulas for less money.

• Laughing out loud every time you hear someone talk about "chemical free" cosmetics.

Speaking of laughing, don't think that just because this book is written by chemists that it's filled with dry, scientific jargon. We're here to educate AND entertain. Don't believe us? Just check out the chapter on bizarre beauty ingredients. (Come on, be honest, aren't you DYING to know if bull semen is really good for your hair?)

Who are the authors?

We're the founders of The Beauty Brains, the #1 beauty science blog, and we've answered thousands of beauty questions over the past 7 years. In addition, we're veteran cosmetic product developers who worked on some of the most popular beauty products in the world. We've written dozens of science articles and books for Cosmetics & Toiletries, Gale Publishing, and the Marcel Dekker company. Our book, Beginning Cosmetic Chemistry is used in several college programs. Trust us, we know what we're talking about.

Perry Romanowski is a writer, cosmetic chemist, Inventor, scientist, instructor, futurologist, and thought leader. He's also the founder of Chemists Corner blog and training program.

Randy Schueller is a writer, former Sr. Director of Hair and Skin Care R&D for Alberto Culver and Unilever and a member of the National Association of Science Writers.

Part 1: Clever Lies the Beauty Companies Tell You

The cosmetic industry does wonderful things for us. It helps our skin stay young looking, it lets us change our hair color when ever we want, and it keeps our armpits from smelling bad. However, even the best intentioned companies can... exaggerate from time to time. And less scrupulous companies have been known to exaggerate a lot! This chapter helps you understand when companies cross that line and over-exaggerate their claims. Understanding when companies are stretching the truth will make you a smarter shopper.

General questions

Are you cheated when companies sell you the same product at different prices?

Glenda's going shopping...My hair is thick, coarse and dry. Which product should I buy, Pantene or Herbal Essences?

It's interesting that you ask about those two products because, as you can tell if you look at the ingredient lists, they are actually the same basic formula. (They are even covered by the same patents). Since a 22 ounce bottle of Pantene sells for about $5.99 while Herbal Essences sells for about $7.99, you're spending $2.00 more for basically the same thing!

Equal ingredients

Take a look at Pantene's Ice Shine conditioner and Herbal Essences' Hydration Conditioner. If you turn the bottles around you'll see that the first five key ingredients are exactly the same:

> *Water, Stearyl Alcohol, Cyclopentasiloxane, Cetyl Alcohol, and Stearamidopropyl Dimethylamine.*

Are these similarities surprising? Not at all considering that P&G (the company that makes Pantene) bought Clairol (the company that makes Herbal Essences.) Shortly after the purchase, P&G converted the Herbal Essences formulas to their Pantene base.

THE BOTTOM LINE

The good news is that Pantene is an excellent conditioner. The bad news is that if you want the performance of Pantene with the color and fragrance of Herbal Essences, it will cost you more! So, since either product will work fine, go with the one that smells the best to you or is least expensive.

4

What does "reduces the appearance of" mean in beauty claims?

Angie asks...I don't understand what it means when companies say that a skin care product "reduces the appearance of" something like brown spots, redness, or wrinkles. It sounds like vague advertising words to me. Is the implication that it doesn't really do anything to physically change the brown spot, etc.?

Essentially it means just what it says – the "appearance" is reduced not necessarily the underlying physical condition. In most cases changing the physical structure of the skin would make the product a drug. Since most of these products are NOT drugs, they have to add the "weasel words" to their claim that make it clear that they are only changing the appearance. Companies have to be careful with the exact wording of their claims to avoid getting into regulatory/legal trouble.

For example, a wrinkle product that temporarily plumps up wrinkles by adding moisture reduces the appearance of wrinkles. Any type of concealer product that covers up redness or age spots reduces their appearance. But after the product is gone the wrinkles remain.

THE BOTTOM LINE
Many cosmetics exaggerate their claims by relying on weasel words like "helps" and "reduces the appearance of." Watch for qualifying terms like this, especially when shopping for expensive products.

How can I tell if an ingredient list is honest?

Terry says...I am a lover of "chemical free" products because they use ingredients grown from our good earth, not cheaply mass produced in a lab so some company can reap the profits. Not all of us have the knowledge to know what goes into our beauty products but, for example, my old A'kin lavender shampoo gives their customers the knowledge. This type of ingredients list makes me feel happy because I know exactly what's in the bottle, some of which are chemical names I cannot even begin to try to pronounce. In my personal opinion I believe that a product should state what percentage of its ingredients are botanically sourced. This puts the power to the consumer.

If you look at the list of ingredients in the shampoo that Terry mentioned (see below) you'll notice that it gives a "natural" source for each item. Presumably, seeing this natural source makes you trust the product more and makes you more inclined to pay a higher price for it. The is a trick known as greenwashing!

You've been greenwashed!
The truth is that there is nothing natural about Cocamidopropyl Hydroxysultaine. The only way you can produce it is to create it in a lab!

The same is true of the following ingredients in this product: glyceryl laurate, lauryl glucoside, sodium citrate, sodium cocoyl glutamate, sodium gluconate, sodium hydroxymethylglycinate, sodium lauroyl sarcosinate, sodium lauryl sulfoacetate.

You are falling for what we call in the business "greenwashing". Every one of these chemicals is synthetically produced in a lab. The starting materials are irrelevant. In fact, these are the same starting materials that the Big Corporations use, they just don't put the parenthetical information on the label. Which, incidentally, in the United States is illegal.

A'kin Lavender Shampoo Ingredients

> *Aqua (purified Australian water*) *BP 2007 standard, citric acid (botanical source), cocamidopropyl hydroxysultaine (from coconut), disodium cocoamphodiacetate (from coconut), glycerin (botanical source), glyceryl laurate (botanical source), lauryl glucoside (from coconut, palm & glucose), sodium citrate (botanical source), sodium cocoyl glutamate (from coconut & sugar cane), sodium gluconate (from GMO free corn), sodium hydroxymethylglycinate, sodium lauroyl sarcosinate (from palm), sodium lauryl sulfoacetate (from palm), sorbitol (from GMO free maize), pelargonium graveolens (geranium) flower oil, rosmarinus officinalis (rosemary) leaf oil, elettaria cardamomum seed oil, lavandula angustifolia (lavender) oil (certified organic), citrus aurantium amara (bitter orange) leaf oil (petitgrain), pogostemon cablin oil*

THE BOTTOM LINE

You can't always take an ingredient list at face value. This is especially true of products from smaller companies, because they are more likely to take chances and exaggerate information than larger companies who are more likely to get caught.

The 10 most misleading cosmetic claims

We were reading some of our latest Twitter updates when we saw another claim about a beauty product being "chemical free." Reading claims like this really bug us because nearly EVERYTHING is a chemical.

There is no such thing as a Chemical Free Sunscreen!!! Zinc Oxide and Titanium Dioxide are CHEMICALS!!

Alright, enough of that. We'll calm down. But it does remind us of all the other misleading cosmetic claims that we see from cosmetic marketers. Here is a list of 10 of the most misleading cosmetic claims that we could find.

What makes a claim misleading?

Before we get to the list, let's define our terms. There are plenty of more egregious claims than the ones on this list, but typically those are direct lies. (e.g. cosmetics that say they will regrow your hair).

The claims listed here are not lies per se; the companies no doubt have supporting tests. However, they are specifically made to mislead consumers.

1. Natural, organic, green, etc.

This claim can mean anything because there is no specific definition for 'natural'. Some companies argue that if an ingredient comes from a natural source then it's natural. They conveniently overlook the fact that they chemically modify it to make it work the way they want it. And 'organic' is not much better. True, there is a USDA organic certification program but it is not required that a cosmetic company follow it to use the 'organic' claim on their products.

Why it is misleading – Companies who use this claim want consumers to believe that the products they produce are "safer" than other cosmetics. Natural / organic / green cosmetics are not safer.

2. Chemical free.

Every cosmetic or personal care product you can buy is made of chemicals. There is no such thing as a 'chemical free' cosmetic. Water is a chemical. Titanium Dioxide is a chemical.

Why it is misleading – It's just wrong. It also is made to imply that the product is "safer" than cosmetics made with chemicals. The products are not safer. This is just wrong.

3. pH balanced

Skin and hair products often advertise themselves as 'pH balanced', as if that is supposed to be some big benefit. What products are sold that are not pH balanced?

Why it is misleading – Companies who make this claim try to imply some superiority over products that are not making this claim. They want consumers to believe that the products will be less irritating and will work better. They won't. Why? Because any decently formulated product will be made in a pH range that is compatible with skin and hair. A consumer will never notice a single difference between a product that is "pH balanced" and one that is just normally formulated.

4. Hypoallergenic

Companies make this claim because they want consumers to believe that their products will not cause allergies. But the FDA looked at this issue in the 1970?s and essentially concluded that the term hypoallergenic has no real meaning, so anyone can make this claim.

Why it is misleading – Hypoallergenic products are not safer or more gentle, even though this is what the claim is meant to imply.

5. "Helps" claim

While it would be illegal to make a claim that a cosmetic product fixes some particular problem directly, it is perfectly fine for companies to claim that the product "helps" fix a problem. Since the word 'help' is sufficiently vague, any product could support a claim that it is helping some condition, whether it is or not.

Why it is misleading – Companies use the qualifier "helps" to be able to make a claim that they want even though they can't support it. For example, when a skin product says "...moisturizes to help strengthen the skin's barriers function..." they really want consumers to think that the skin's barrier function will be strengthened. However, they don't have any evidence that the product will do this. Adding the word 'helps' lets them make the claim without having to have the evidence.

6. Patented formula

Companies love to claim 'patented' or 'unique' or 'exclusive' formula. What they want consumers to believe is that the formula is somehow special and will work better than competitors.

Why this is misleading – It's relatively easy to find some way to patent a formula, but that doesn't mean the patent will somehow make the product a superior personal care product. Often cosmetic patents are just technicalities that made it past a naive patent examiner. Typically, the patent has nothing to do with how well the formula performs.

7. Makes hair stronger

This is a pet peeve of ours. Products that claim to make hair stronger do not make hair stronger. What they really do is make hair less prone to breakage when it is being combed. This isn't hair strength, it's conditioning.

Why this is misleading – If you test the strength of hair with a tensile test or other force measuring device, you will discover that hair is not actually stronger. But consumers are meant to believe that hair becomes stronger even though it doesn't.

8. Boosts collagen production

You find this claim in lots of cosmetic products.

Why it is misleading – If the product actually increased the amount of collagen your skin produced, it would be a mislabeled drug. Cosmetics are not allowed to have a significant impact on your skin metabolism.

9. Reduces the appearance of wrinkles

Most any anti-aging product is going to make this claim and it's very likely true. However, the message that consumers get from this claim is different than the words that are written and marketers know this.

Why it is misleading – While the product is only reducing the "appearance" of wrinkles, consumers read that and believe that the product will somehow get rid of wrinkles. It won't. Almost no cosmetic skin cream is going to get rid of wrinkles. They might make wrinkles look less obvious, but this isn't what consumers think when they read a claim like that.

10. Proven formula

The term proven is powerful in the consumer's mind, even though it doesn't have to mean much of anything.

Why it is misleading – Marketers know that the term 'proven' automatically makes consumers think that the product works. And maybe it does work, but it almost never works in the way (or to the extent) that consumers will think it works. This is why it is a misleading claim.

Claims and the cosmetic chemist

Unfortunately, cosmetic companies have to make misleading claims, because this is what consumers respond to. There are certainly some claims that are more egregious than others, but as a cosmetic chemist you should be able to recognize those and help your marketing department find ways to make non-misleading claims. It's not easy, but someone should be doing it.

Beauty companies must think we're stupid

We know that beauty companies have to be increasingly creative with their claims and advertising in order to break through the clutter and entice us to buy their products. But sometimes we're offended when they make ridiculous scientific-sounding claims. Are they just being "cute", or do they really think we're stupid enough to believe whatever they tell us? Maybe it's just us, but when we saw these three new products we had to cringe a little bit, because they seem to disrespect our intelligence.

Millionize your lashes

First is Voluminous Million Lashes mascara, which claims it will "millionize your lashes." We don't really know what that means, but it kind of creeps us out. We like the idea of thick long lashes, but we're not sure we want millions of them sticking out from all over our eyes. Or perhaps they mean their product will make our normal lashes 1 million times thicker. Since on average a human hair is about 0.002 inches in diameter, increasing the size by 1 million times would make each eyelash approximately 167 feet in diameter. Maybe it's just us, but we don't find that very appealing.

DNA Advantage

Next is Revlon's new DNA makeup. It contains something called "DNA Advantage tm." We have no idea what this is, but clearly this product is better than others on the market because it's SHAPED LIKE THE DNA DOUBLE HELIX. Watson and Crick would be proud.

Reacts to light and pH

Finally there is the Physician's Formula entry into the "this product changes color to match your skin tone, honest it does" category. This time, in addition to pH control, this product is also activated by light to give you the "perfect bronze glow." Of course it's activated by light - you can't see your foundation in the dark!

THE BOTTOM LINE

Creative, compelling claims are one thing. Ridiculous statements that insult our intelligence are another!

What are "Active" ingredients?

Kelly inquires...You often mention "active ingredients" – what are they and which are the "non-active" ingredients?

We love this question, even though there is no simple, straightforward answer. While other cosmetic chemists may have their own definitions, we like to think that you can break all beauty product ingredients down into five basic categories:

5 Types of Cosmetic Ingredients
Active ingredients: They deliver the promise of the product.
Of course, the type of activity varies widely. We guess the "truest" active ingredients are those specified as drugs by the appropriate governing body. So UV absorbers in sunscreens, benzoyl peroxide in anti-acne creams, and fluoride in toothpaste are all REALLY active.

But even the surfactants used in a shampoo or body wash are active by our definition – they are responsible for getting your hair or skin clean, which is the basic promise of the product. The same thing goes for the silicones in a hair conditioner, the colorants in a mascara, or the polymers in a hairspray. If the ingredient is essential to making the product work, then it is "active."

Base ingredients: They form the delivery vehicle for the active ingredients.

Active ingredients are rarely used by themselves in a 100% concentrated form. There's usually an optimal use level for ingredients to ensure they do their job. Therefore the actives have to be "diluted" with something. That something may be as simple as water or as complex as a cream or lotion base or an aerosol spray. It may take dozens of ingredients to form the "base" of the product. Solvents, like water and alcohol, and emulsifiers, to help oils and water mix together, are among the most common types of base ingredients.

Control ingredients: They ensure the product stays within acceptable parameters.

Gums and polymers are used to stabilize emulsions, acids and bases are used to balance pH, polyols are used to maintain texture after freezing, and preservatives are used to protect against microbial contamination. These are just a few examples of control agents that help maintain the quality of the product.

Aesthetic agents: They improve the product's sensory characteristics.

The look and smell are important parts of almost every cosmetic product, which is why you'll see colorants and fragrance used so frequently. You might even see "glitter" particles added.

Featured ingredients: They are added to increase consumer appeal.

These ingredients are also called pixie dust, fairy dust, marketing ingredients and a few other names. These are truly "inactive" because they're added ONLY because they look good as part of the label. They serve no function other than to attract consumers' attention. These ingredients include botanicals, vitamins and minerals, (some) proteins and just about anything else "natural." You can easily spot these ingredients, because they are often incorporated into the product name (Sun-kissed Raspberry Shampoo) or placed on the front label (lotion with jojoba oil).

THE BOTTOM LINE
You can be a smarter beauty shopper by understanding which ingredients are truly active and which ones are there just to make the product look good.

Why do companies sell different quality brands?

Amy asks...I recently saw a list of which companies own which brands of cosmetics. For example – L'Oreal owns Maybelline, Lancome, L'Oreal, Shu Uemura, etc...So why is it that these brands make such different quality products? They're obviously not competitors, though they are seen like that through the general public's eyes. Is it just the whole marketing scheme?

It's fascinating to find out which companies really own your favorite brands. It can also help you save money!

It's a brand-eat-brand world
There are several reasons that a company could own multiple brands with different levels of quality. One reason is that as part of their growth strategy companies strive to acquire other companies or brands. That's a quick way to grow a business, and through these acquisitions the companies end up with a patchwork quilt of multiple brands.

Also, many companies also find it desirable to sell products at different price points. That's why they may have a budget brand sold in dollar stores, a medium priced brand sold in drug stores, and a prestige brand sold in department stores. This strategy allows them to market products to a broader audience through more outlets. (Of course, the profit margins are very different across these different price points!)

THE BOTTOM LINE
If you're savvy about which companies own which brands, you can look at the ingredient lists on products made by the same company. Sometimes you'll find that the cheaper brand uses the same ingredients as the more expensive one!

Why "Chemical Free" claims are harmful

The claim "chemical free" really bugs us and we really wish marketers, the media, and everyone else would stop using it. Almost nothing is "chemical free"!!

Our latest irritation with the claim was from an article published on the Times Free Press website titled "Chemical free ways to clean your home." The author recommends "chemical free" products like Vinegar, Salt, Baking Soda, Lemon Juice and Castile Soap.

What!?

Has this reporter ever taken a chemistry class?

Vinegar is Acetic Acid...a chemical

Kosher salt is Sodium Chloride...a chemical

Baking soda is Sodium Bicarbonate...a chemical

Lemon Juice is mostly Citric Acid...another chemical

Ugh!

Why, why, why would someone publish such nonsense? What do they even mean when they say "chemical free"? It certainly can't literally mean chemical free.

Insidious Chemical Free

Our complaints about chemical free are more than just semantics. This insidious claim has a number of negatives associated with it. And these will be problems for cosmetic chemists and formulators who want to produce safe, functional, and excellent products. Here are the primary problems with chemical free.

1. Chemical free is inaccurate. Almost nothing is chemical free. All matter is made up of chemicals (elements). And all products are made up of matter. Water is a chemical (2 parts Hydrogen, 1 part Oxygen). Vinegar is a chemical. The only things that are not chemical are things like light, electricity, magnetism, or subatomic particles.

These are unlikely to be the composition of your "chemical free" cosmetic or cleaning product.

2. Chemical free is deceptive and misleading. This is the most significant problem with the chemical free claim. It is used when the marketer wants to say "this product is safer than other products". The implication is that "chemical free" products are safer than "chemical containing" products. Of course, since every product contains chemicals, the claim is a lie. The implication that a "chemical free" product is safer is also a lie. "Chemical free" cosmetics are not demonstrably safer than ones that don't claim "chemical free". It's a lie! Consumers are being duped. We don't know why these claims are allowed, especially when they are false advertising.

Consumers deserve accuracy in advertising and they should not be lied to. There is no such thing as a chemical free cosmetic and these claims of "chemical free" sunscreens are complete fabrications!

These claims are spreading scientific ignorance and leading to the erosion of critical thinking among the general population. There really should be a law or, at the very least, people who make inaccurate "chemical free" claims should be publicly flogged. Metaphorically of course.

Do beauty companies ever get caught lying?

Carol's question..."If so many cosmetics claims are untrue, how can beauty companies get away with lying to us?"

The answer is that they don't always get away with lying. Case in point:

Aloe Vera Angst
FDA raps aloe vera company for violating regulatory Act By Michelle Yeomans , 12-Jul-2012

The Set-N-Me-Free Aloe Vera company got their hand slapped by the FDA for making unsupported drug claims for their aloe vera-based line of products (including 'Aloe Milk Moisturizing', 'Aloe Moisture Cream', 'Day-Night Emollients', 'Moisturizing Aloe Lotion' and 'Aloe Comfrey Gel'.)

What was the problem?
The company apparently claimed the following about their products...

Moisturizing Aloe Lotion can help "renew skin flexibility by making regeneration of skin cells occur faster."

Day-Night Emollient contained "natural source of cancer-fighting laetryl lipids"

and that their aloe ingredient is capable of "similar anti-inflammatory properties similar to that of a steroid."

Since all these claims would involve affecting the physiology of the body, they are legally drug claims. This violation falls under section 201(g)(1)(B) and/or 201(g)(1)(C) of the Federal Food, Drug, and Cosmetic Act. (But we're sure you knew that already.)

What's the FDA going to do?
Since these are misbranded drugs (i.e., products that make drug claims without following the proper drug labeling laws) the FDA has asked the company to change their claims (on websites, labels, and promotional materials) to ensure they do not violate the law. If the

company does not enact appropriate changes, the FDA can bring "regulatory action." Oooooh, we're scared.

THE BOTTOM LINE

You may not always realize it, but there are penalties when cosmetic companies stretch the truth too much. If you'd like to see more examples of how the FDA takes action against misleading advertising by beauty companies, you should subscribe to the newsfeed for CosmeticsDesign.com

Avoid high priced hype by learning how to spot quackery

There are thousands of beauty companies out there selling "hope in a bottle." Too many times they try to entice you to spend your hard-earned money by exaggerating what their products can really do. If you can learn to spot exaggerated claims you'll be a smarter shopper.

A list of their Red Flags of Quackery.
Be wary of products that use any of these phrases or claims in their advertising, because they might just be out to get your money.

1. Testimonials

2. "Helps your body"

3. Celebrity Doctor

4. Ancient Wisdom

5. Secret/Conspiracy

6. "Buy my book"

7. "Miracle ingredient"

8. Non-MD Doctor

9. "Natural"

10. "Quantum"

11. "Toxins"

12. "Energy"

13. "Magnets"

14. Hostility to criticism

15. "Western Medicine"

THE BOTTOM LINE

Having a skeptical mindset is the best way to prevent yourself from wasting money on over-priced and over-hyped products. Before purchasing a cosmetic that uses any of these red flags, do some research first!

How can I find another version of my favorite product?

Nancy needs to know...The leave-in conditioner "It's a 10" was recommended to me by my stylist to cut down on split ends and frizz. I have fine hair and even when its clean and brushed/combed tends to look messy, and it tangles very easily. I have been using the "It's a 10" leave-in for the last few weeks every time I shampoo my hair and have been very happy with the results. My problem, I HATE the way it smells. It's not that the scent is a bad one, I just personally don't like it. Is there a similar product that has a different or no scent?

You came to the right place, Nancy. Here's our secret for finding similar products.

First, here are the ingredients for the product you asked about:

> Water, Cetearyl Alcohol, Behentrimonium Chloride, Menthylparaben, Propylparaben, Propylene Glycol, Panthenol, Cyclomethicone, Silk Amino Acids, Heli Anthus Annuus, Sunflower Seed Extract, Camellia Sinensis Leaf Extract, Quaternium-80, Fragrance, Citric Acid, Methylchloroisothiazaolinone and Methylisothiazolinone.

How to find similar products:
Search online (or look in stores) for other leave-in sprays.

Check the ingredient list to make sure it's water based (water should be the first ingredient.)

Then look for "Behentrimonium Chloride" in the first 3 or 4 ingredients. That means the product should be pretty similar.

Look for "Cyclomethicone" after the first 5 ingredients. That means it's even closer.

Look for Quaternium-80 after that. If the product you find has all three of these ingredients, it should be VERY similar.

Smell the product before you buy it so you know you like the fragrance!

THE BOTTOM LINE

We can't guarantee this approach will find an exact duplicate of the "It's a 10" product, but it should help you narrow down your choices and increase the likelihood that you'll find something you'll like. (You might even be able to save some money!) You can use this same general approach of matching the first five ingredients for almost any product.

Has this antibacterial soap website ignored science?

We like the Personal Care Products Council (aka the PCPC) and believe that for the most part they do an excellent job of ensuring that our cosmetic products are safe and effective. The cosmetic industry is not interested in poisoning its consumers, and the PCPC helps prevent a waste of time and effort that the FDA would have to expend if it had to enforce more regulation. We also think the INCI is an excellent resource for all people interested in cosmetics.

However, the PCPC is not perfect and the launch of their recent website FightGermsNow.com is a good reminder.

The good

The goal of the website is laudable. They aim to be the the official source on antibacterial hygiene products. This is great. Consumers, scientists, and regulators could use a site like this. We're all for giving people information, and fighting germs is certainly important. We also like the way they have a tab for the relevant regulations with links to the proper governmental agencies. Finally, we like the safety information they provide. No doubt, antibacterial products are safe to use (at least for the user).

The bad

After that, it goes downhill for us. They have a tab of 'Surveys' which lists people's attitudes about antibacterial products. This is fine enough, but we don't exactly understand why it is useful. Perhaps regulators might find it interesting. But it seems to us to just be a measure of how well people are responding to the marketing efforts of companies that sell antibacterial soaps. It is also presented in a way that suggests that antibacterial soaps are good because the majority of people use them and find them useful.

We have to say that whether people find them useful or not is relevant to whether they are actually useful. This is the kind of thing you would see in a marketing effort for antibacterial soap rather than in a scientific website about it.

The ugly
While the survey tab is just bad, the really ugly stuff is the things included under the "Facts" and "Science" tabs. These things are not Facts and the Science is not presented as Science.

Let's look at the Facts and Science pages.

One claim they make is that

> "Using personal cleaning products that contain an active anti-bacterial or antimicrobial ingredient helps to provide extra protection against germs that cause many common illnesses (e.g. skin infections, food poisoning, intestinal illnesses)."

We're not sure there is good evidence for this. Certainly not good enough evidence to call it a fact.

This is on the antibacterial soap page but then again on the Science page.

> "Antibacterial hand washes have been shown to reduce the numbers of germs on the skin to a greater extent than washing with plain soap"

We found this strange, because we remember reading this report that Antibacterial soap is not better than regular soap. Perhaps there was another study that countered the claims made by this study.

What we appreciate about the FightGermsNow website is that they provide links to studies to support their claim. This is good. This is science. Unfortunately, the links they provided do not support what they are claiming as FACT.

Analysis of FACTS
For example, in support of "FACT: Antibacterial hand soaps provide greater germ-fighting protection than regular soap and water", they list a scientific model and expert panel review as evidence to support the fact.

STRIKE 1 – Models and expert opinions are good predictions but they don't make something a FACT.

The next study they list is Alternative hand contamination technique to compare the activities of antimicrobial and non-antimicrobial soaps under different test conditions

They list the abstract, but upon further investigation, they REMOVED a crucial sentence in the abstract which disputes what they list as a FACT!

The website writes "Antimicrobial hand soaps provide a greater bacterial reduction than non-antimicrobial soaps. Confounding factors, such as compliance, soap volume, and wash time, may all influence the outcomes of studies."

But the full abstract says "Antimicrobial hand soaps provide a greater bacterial reduction than non-antimicrobial soaps. However, the link between greater bacterial reduction and a reduction of disease has not been definitively demonstrated. Confounding factors, such as compliance, soap volume, and wash time, may all influence the outcomes of studies. "

STRIKE 2 – Leaving out statements that don't support your fact is a clear manipulation.

Then another study they provide as support for their fact is Comparative efficacy of hand hygiene agents in the reduction of bacteria and viruses

Somehow they didn't read the whole conclusion, because it clearly states that "Effective hand hygiene for high levels of viral contamination with a nonenveloped virus was best achieved by physical removal with a non-antimicrobial soap or tap water alone."

STRIKE 3 – Ignoring facts that don't support your claim is wrong

THE BOTTOM LINE

Like we said, we're fans of the PCPC and believe that overall they do a great job. But when they get into the business of marketing one technology over another, we think they've gone too far. And with this FightGermsNow website, they certainly strain their credibility as an unbiased, science-based organization.

Skin care/makeup questions

Are pH-balanced products better?

Lana longs to learn...Should I only buy skin products that are pH-balanced?

We've always maintained that pH balanced skin care products are just marketing hype, because the skin's natural pH resets itself within as little as 15 minutes after applying lotion. But as good scientists, we're always willing to change our minds when new evidence is presented. In this particular case, new evidence has come in the form of an article written by the BeautyBrains' favorite dermatologist, Zoe Diana Draelos, M.D. Should we change our opinion that pH balance is bunk? Read on to find out.

Acid reign?

In her article on Modernmedicine.com (http://thebeautybrains.com/W9hX8), Dr. Draelos points out that while the idea of pH-balanced products began as a "marketing strategy" for products that have a neutral pH, there may actually be a benefit to using products that have a pH balance on the acidic side of the scale.

That's because relatively new research shows that if the skin has trouble maintaining its naturally acidic pH (known as the acid mantle), then it may be more susceptible to certain diseases caused by bacterial growth. Therefore, products around pH 4 can help reduce bacterial colonization of the skin. However, the good doctor also points out that "products that are pH-balanced may offer some benefit in patients with skin disease." (Emphasis ours.) In other words, if you have healthy skin you shouldn't have a problem using products with a "regular" pH.

So while we're in full agreement with the expert assessment that in some special circumstances the pH of the product can make a difference, we maintain our stance that in the general case, pH balance is more hyperbole than healthy.

THE BOTTOM LINE

Unless you have a skin disease, you don't need to waste your money on products that expect you to pay more just because of their pH.

Special benefits of mineral makeup

We were interviewed by a writer for WebMD who asked questions about mineral makeup. From an ingredient perspective, mineral makeup is all over the place. Some companies market products that are truly based exclusively on minerals. But others sell mineral makeup that includes ingredients that are NOT minerals like oils and non-mineral colorants.

We're curious what your beliefs about mineral makeup are (because we're curious to see how effective the marketing behind these products has been.) So, we asked the Beauty Brains Forum to share their beliefs about mineral makeup. Here is what they had to say...

Less irritating

I use it because it's less occlusive than liquid makeup and it does not contain irritants (like chemical sunscreens) that aggravate my rosacea. But the same could be said for any powder makeup. -SF

I think most consumers would agree with me in that they have come to know "mineral" as meaning a product containing natural, hypo-allergenic ingredients, as opposed to old-fashioned powders that may still contain skin-irritating synthetic ingredients. -JE

Better oil control

I use powder mineral makeup, but mostly just because it IS powder and on my oily skin that works better. A definite plus is that it doesn't break my skin out. That being said, it doesn't work for me at all unless I use a primer under it. Go figure. -LG

The only benefit with mineral makeup I find is my forehead tends to be less shiny. I use liquid mineral makeup, then put powder over that. Otherwise, it's just the same, and in some cases worse, as non-mineral. In the end, I think it's a lot of hype. If it wasn't for the fact that an hour after washing my forehead is shiny enough to signal airplanes at night, I wouldn't bother with mineral makeup at all. -JS

Convenience
Oh and another reason…. it is powder and therefore does not have to fit into the 3-1-1 bag for travel! -LG

Non-allergenic
Well…I use mineral make up, because it is actually the only make-up that doesn't contain ingredients that I am allergic to… But if I didn't have any allergies I would go for all the 'normal' make up. I don't use it simply because it claims to better for the environment or that it would be non-toxic. Those claims do not sound very valid to me. So yes, I am very happy with mineral make-up, because it makes it possible for me to wear make-up (I could not live without…) without getting scary allergic reactions. -K

Better coverage
I just like the coverage I get…I think I can get the same coverage with regular powder makeup, but honestly I haven't really tried. Almost every brand now makes some kind of mineral claim on their powder makeups that I haven't noticed any powders without it! So that's why I continue to use it. -LM

Liquid foundation was making my skin dry, and I never really got the same finish each time, and that's in any texture very runny, thick or mousse (the mousse was a disaster and the blush too!). The powder oddly stays all day, and it also gives a more natural finish. They had just the perfect shades of eyeshadow that I'd been looking for, and it just so happened that it stays all day. -BC

Compelling Advertising
Marketing mind games was definitely part of the reason I decided to try some… cute name, pretty website, pretty product descriptions, haha, but hey, the products work. It wasn't about it being mineral, it was just they had such good reviews and I was sick of horrible cakey skin.-BC

I admit, I started using mineral powder makeup because I saw a commercial of the "pioneer" brand on tv and thought it was a miracle. I totally bought into the "safety" aspect, and the "amazing coverage" messages. That was about 5 years ago...Now that I am Beauty Brains savvy, I don't care whether it has minerals or not. -LM

THE BOTTOM LINE

There are no clear rules about what is and isn't a mineral makeup. Therefore you should be careful not to spend more money on products that claim to contain pure minerals unless you've done your research first.

Do facial masks remove toxins?

Peggy has a point...If you have not tried the Rare Earth skincare line yet, this is a great time to try it. As a gal with oily skin who is not a fan of her pores, this product line targets them to pull all the toxins and gunk out of your pores. What's not to love?

While we agree that Kiehl's makes great products, "what's not to love" is the price! Their products always seem overpriced to us. Is there a way to get the same benefits for less money?

(We'd be remiss if we didn't point out that masks can help remove dead skins cells but they don't really pull "toxins" out of your skin or blood. That's what your liver is for!)

Kiehl's Rare Earth Ingredients ($22 for 5 oz.)

Water, Kaolin, Bentonite, Glycerin, Propylene Glycol, CI 77891, Zea mays, Phenoxyethanol, Polysorbate 80, Tocopherol Methylparaben Lecithin Retinyl Palmitate, Allantoin, acetyl methionine, Serica, Avena sativa, Prunus armeniaca, Persea gratissima, Triticum Vulgare, Guaiazulene, TBHQ, aloe barbadensis leaf extract.

Cautious clay

The most important ingredients in facial masks are the clays that produce the drying, tightening sensation. There are two basic types, and Kiehl's has them both: Kaolin clay (aka China clay or White clay) is very mild and is used for both sensitive skin and dry skin. It is good for use in masks because it does not expand with increasing water content. However, using too much Kaolin can make the product feel gritty.

Bentonite clay (a combination of montmorillonite and volcanic ash) is very absorbent and is best suited for oily skin. It doesn't dissolve in water, but it will absorb enough to swell to about eight times its weight. However, large amounts of Bentonite will make the mask take longer to dry. In small quantities it helps make the mask more elastic.

The best mask formulas use a blend of both of these ingredients.

Queen Helene Mint Julep Masque Ingredients ($6.99 for 12 oz.)

> *Water, Kaolin, Bentonite (CI 77004), Glycerin, Zinc Oxide, Propylene Glycol, Sulfur, Chromium Oxide Green (CI#77288), Fragrance (Parfum), Phenoxyethanol, Methylparaben.*

As you can see, both products have a blend of Kaolin and Bentonite. But Kiehl's is almost 9 times more expensive than Queen Helene! At that price, the best use for this product may be to wear it as a face mask when you rob a bank so you can afford to buy more. (Just kiddin', kind of.) But seriously, at that price, the cheaper alternatives, like Queen Helene, are at least worth a look.

THE BOTTOM LINE
Once again, you can save money by comparing the first five items on the ingredient lists of two products.

Can cosmetics really change color to match your skin?

Dana asks...Products like Smashbox O-Glow Blush and Jemma Kidd Lip Gloss claim to to change color to match your skin tone or even match your mood. Is that really possible? Can cosmetics somehow detect your natural skin tone or even your emotional state and then adjust their color to match?

The answer is no. This beauty myth is quite popular, but it's simply not true. Here's how color changing products REALLY work.

3 types of color-changing chemistry
1. Ingredients that change color with pH/solubility

Most of the products that we see that make these claims use this approach. The main ingredient that provides the effect is a colorant known as "Red 27," a red dye which is colorless when dissolved in a waterless base. When it comes in contact with moisture, the change in solubility and pH causes the dye to turn bright pink. The product appears to change with your personal chemistry because the color changes when it comes in contact with moisture that comes from your skin, or even just the humidity in the air. Red 27 can be used in powdered cosmetics, waxy sticks, and gels.

Example products that use Red 27:

Stila Custom Color Blush

Smashbox O-Glow Blush

DuWop Personal Color Changing Lipstick

2. Encapsulated colors

Some products use colorants that are coated with waxy or gel-like ingredients and suspended in an uncolored base. When the product is rubbed into your skin the friction breaks open the dye capsules, releasing the color. The product appears to change with your personal chemistry because the more your rub in the color, the more is released. Encapsulated colors work best in cream and powder based products.

Example product that uses encapsulated colors:

Intuitive Blend Shade Adjusting Foundation by Wet n' Wild

3. Skin protein reaction

Products that provide a "natural tan glow" work by using an ingredient called "dihydroxyacetone" or DHA. This chemical reacts with the keratin protein in the upper layers of your skin, staining them a light orangish-brown color. The product appears to change with your personal chemistry because it uses low levels of DHA that provides a very gradual change in skin color. The more you use, the more pronounced the "glow" effect is.

Example product that uses a skin protein reaction:

Jergen's Natural Glow

Does age, skin color, or other factors affect how they work?
As described above, the chemistry involved in the color change has little to do with a woman's individual skin chemistry. However, the color of her skin will have a significant effect on the appearance of the cosmetic color. As your skin color changes (either with age or sun exposure) the color of these cosmetics could look different. This is not an issue for lip products since the skin on your lips doesn't change with age or sun exposure.

Contraindications: Who should not use them?
None of the chemistries we've seen used in these products have any special contraindications. Of course, as with any cosmetic, you may be sensitive to specific ingredients that could cause an allergic reaction. If this occurs, you should discontinue using the product as soon as you notice any warning signs, such as redness or irritation.

THE BOTTOM LINE

While it's true that cosmetics can change color, the idea that they can match your mood is a myth. Don't be fooled into wasting money on products like this.

Do Frownies really fight wrinkles?

Helen asks...Are Frownies really a Hollywood beauty secret? Do they help to smooth forehead lines and creases between your eyebrows (especially if someone has a habit of scrunching eyebrows)?

This question has come up from several of our readers. Lucy, for example, asked, "Can using a patch to relax muscles while sleeping reduce wrinkles?" The answer comes from understanding the underlying role of muscles in facial wrinkles (pun intended). But first let's look at how Frownies are supposed to work.

What are Frownies?

Frownies have been around since the late 1800?s, and they are allegedly used by Hollywood's elite to secretly fight wrinkles. These adhesive strips are applied between the eyes, across the forehead, and at the corners of the eyes and mouth. According to their website, the strips "gently re-educate the underlying muscles to assume their correct, relaxed and natural appearance." They form a "splint" that holds the top layer of the skin in place so skin cells in the underlying layers can "reposition themselves," thus removing the wrinkle.

Do Frownies really remove wrinkles?

As Helen asked, can you remove wrinkles by "splinting" the skin? According to the opinions of the dermatologists that we've read the answer is "not so much" because muscle activity is not really the cause of wrinkles. In an interview on St. John Providence.org (http://thebeautybrains.com/sLBET), Dr Fedok, director of facial plastic and reconstructive surgery at Pennsylvania State University, says "It's more due to damage from the sun." That's because over time UV radiation breaks down elastin and collagen, the components of the skin that give it structural integrity. This loss of structure is the real cause of wrinkles, and manipulating the underlying muscles (either relaxing them or exercising them) won't restore the collagen and elastin. In the same article, another dermatologist, Dr. Basler of the American Academy of Dermatology, says "The only thing that's going to push those wrinkles out is if you increase the volume of your face, like blowing air into a balloon." The good doctor Fedok also points out that gravity causes wrinkles by pulling on the connective ligament-like tissues that hold facial fat pads in place. Again, Frownies won't undo the effect of gravity on stretched ligaments.

OK, what about preventing wrinkles?

When it comes to Frownies, an ounce of prevention may be worth a pound of cure. At least theoretically. Dr. Fedok points out that some wrinkles, like laugh lines, can be caused by exaggerated facial expressions that eventually create changes in skin structure. If that's the case, it's plausible that, if worn long enough, Frownies could help prevent those wrinkles by helping you relax the muscles associated with those "exaggerated facial expressions." Maybe that explains why people seem to love these things (at least if you can trust the overwhelming positive reviews on sites like drugstore.com.) Of course, without controlled studies, we'll never know if there is a real benefit to Frownies, or if the positive impression is just a halo effect. (And believe us, we looked for definitive studies and could find none.)

THE BOTTOM LINE

Based on input from dermatologists, it appears unlikely that Frownies are able to reverse wrinkles. However, they may be able to prevent some wrinkles that are formed by repetitive facial expressions.

Can nail polish really be healthy?

KP asks...Can nail polish, like from Remedy Nails, be "healthy"? Is their claim that they have the most unique polish on the market true?

It's tough to answer a question like this without a standard definition of what "healthy" means.

Healthy polish?
We had trouble finding much information about how Remedy Nails claims to be so healthy and unique, so we wrote to the company asking for an explanation. Unfortunately, they have not responded. So, we can't really tell for sure how they support their claims. In our humble opinion, it all depends on how you define "healthy." Having worked in the beauty industry for many years, we can speculate how a company might respond when asked "What does healthy mean?"

Definition 1: Free from damage (that negatively affects appearance)
Example: Healthy looking nails.

Comment: Claims related to appearance are almost always easily substantiated.

Definition 2: Free from disease
Example: Fights nail fungus.

Comment: This would be a drug claim, so we doubt Remedy Nails would use such as approach - unless, of course, they are selling a drug product.

Definition 3: Improved quality
Example: Stronger nails, longer lasting color, etc.

Comment: This is a gray area. Nail strengtheners can also cause brittleness. Is that really healthier? Many people would say no.

Definition 4: Less dangerous side effects, less toxic
Example: No harmful solvents.

Comment: We've written about the dangers of breathing nail polish, and there is certainly reason for concern about neurotoxicity. Water-based polishes could "healthier" in this regard. Perhaps this is Remedy's approach? If so, do they provide the same quality polish as solvent-based systems? If not, you have to ask yourself: how much are you willing to give up to get a "healthier" product?

THE BOTTOM LINE

As you can see from these examples, "healthy" is a very subjective claim that is open to interpretation. It would be interesting to see how Remedy Nails defines "healthy" for their products.

How can I tell I'm using enough antioxidants?

Fay asks...I also use olive oil as a facial moisturizer. Does this provide sufficient antioxidant protection?

Assessing how much antioxidant protection you need is a more difficult question to answer than you might imagine. We just read a great article by one of our favorite dermatologists, Zoe Diana Draelos, (http://thebeautybrains.com/5pTwn) that explains the difficulty in measuring antioxidant efficacy under real life conditions. But first we'll provide a little background.

Why are antioxidants important?
Your skin (and other body tissues) can contain molecules known as free radicals – these are harmful substances that contain an unpaired electron. When they're in pairs, electrons are "balanced" and don't pose a problem. But the "loose" electron in free radicals can attack cells in the body and cause all kinds of havoc. That's where antioxidants come to the rescue: they can stabilize the free radical either by donating an electron to it or by neutralizing it. Problem solved!

Do antioxidants work in skincare?
Unfortunately, it's not easy to tell how well antioxidants really work. In her article, Dr. Draelos points out the two key problems with understanding how many antioxidants you really need: With ingested antioxidants it's hard to know the proper dose. (For example, she says that questions have been raised on whether or not high doses of vitamin C are really helping your body or just creating "expensive urine.")

Second, for topical products (antioxidant creams and lotions), it's hard to prevent the antioxidant ingredient from being "used up" by the environmental oxygen when they are applied to the skin. The truth is, scientists don't know how well either of these antioxidant approaches really work.

Tough to measure

Why are the real life effects of antioxidants so unknown? Because, while there are laboratory ways to measure the effect at the cellular level, scientists have very limited tools to measure the real life effects of antioxidants. Dr. Draelos says the only currently viable method of measuring antioxidant performance on skin is a test called "the sunburn cell assay." This test involves taking a samples of skin tissue with and without antioxidants of people with a special skin type who have been exposed to UV rays. The effect of the antioxidant can be determined by counting the number of sunburned cells. While it's a very crude method, it's the best that exists right now. Needless to say, not many companies go to the trouble of testing their products to this extent. That's why it's really hard to answer your question.

THE BOTTOM LINE

We agree with Dr. Draelos' point that antioxidants are an important part of a sun-protective program, but you should realize that claims around the efficacy of any specific antioxidants are controversial.

Are tinted moisturizers and foundation just the same thing?

Nicki asks… I've read in so many magazines that have said tinted moisturizers are better than foundation on the skin. What exactly is the difference between tinted moisturizers and liquid foundation apart from the fact that tinted moisturizers is lighter? I've also heard from some friends that tinted moisturizers are bad for your skin. So are tinted moisturizers good or bad?

Elizabeth Arden makes both kinds of products, so let's look at the ingredients in their Sheer Lights Illuminating Tinted Moisturizer and Bare Perfection Flawless Finish Foundation as an example. We won't reprint all of the ingredients here, but you can find them on Drugstore.com.

Similar yet different

Both products contain sunscreens as active ingredients. They both use water as a solvent and they both contain mixtures of humectants (chemicals that bind water to skin) and emollients (oily chemicals that smooth skin and create a moisture barrier). Since these are emulsion-type products, they both use surfactants that keep the water- and oil-soluble ingredients mixed together in a creamy base. Of course, they both contain preservatives and ingredients to control the thickness and pH. And, since both are designed to give your skin a bit of color, they contain pigments. Specifically, they both use iron oxides and titanium dioxide.

They sound pretty similar, don't they? They are similar, but not identical. How are they different? Well, the amount of color they contain will vary and so will the consistency of the products. And the moisturizer version appears to have more humectants, so we'd guess it will bind water to your skin better. But overall, they both are basically delivery vehicles for skin tinting pigments.

Given the similarities, it's hard to imagine why one product would be "bad" for you and the other wouldn't. Now, if you have very dry skin, you may prefer the moisturizing version. And likewise if your skin is oily, you might want to use the lighter version. But this isn't a case of "good" versus "bad." It's more about finding what you like.

THE BOTTOM LINE

Tinted moisturizers and foundations may look and feel different, but ultimately they function the same way. In case you didn't realize, the beauty industry often takes similar products and makes them sound very different. There's nothing wrong with that, as long as they're honest about the products' benefits. You'll have to experiment with different products to cut through all this hype and and find the one that's right for you.

Are there really food grade cosmetics?

MB asks...I noticed in the comment section of the blog that someone provided a link to her site where she sells organic cosmetics. Is it really possible for cosmetics to meet food grade standards?

It's possible to make food grade cosmetics, but that doesn't mean it's possible to make good food grade cosmetics.

What standards do we measure natural products by?

Can you make a food grade cosmetic? Sure, you can slap almost any ingredients together and call them a cosmetic. Just mash up an avocado with some wheat germ oil and smear it on your face. It will certainly hydrate your skin, but will it FEEL like a moisturizer should? I think the question should be: "Can you make a food grade (or natural) cosmetic that's of comparable quality to a "regular" cosmetic?" That's where it gets a bit tricky, because in many cases it's difficult, if not impossible, for truly natural ingredients to provide the same level of performance as a synthetic ingredients that have been specifically engineered to deliver a desired benefit. That doesn't mean natural products are bad, it just means you should expect them to be different. And, you need to ask yourself if this difference is acceptable and worth paying more for.

Let's look at two examples from the website in question (organicglow.com) and assess how well they would be expected to perform based on their ingredients. For the sake of discussion, we'll look at two hair care products: shampoo and a hair gel.

Miessence Dessert Flower Shampoo Ingredients

Certified Organic Aloe Barbadensis (aloe vera) Leaf Juice, Coco Glucoside , Yucca Schidigera Extract, D-panthenol (pro-vitamin B5), Non-GMO Xanthan Gum, Citrus Aurantium Amara (bitter orange) Fruit Extract, Certified Organic Helianthus Annuus (sunflower) Seed Oil, Certified Organic Citrus Aurantifolia (lime) Essential Oil, Citric Acid. Certified Organic Persea Gratissima (avocado) Fruit Oil, Certified Organic Equisetum Arvense (horsetail) Extract, Certified Organic Urtica Dioica (nettle) Extract, Certified Organic Arctium Lappa (burdock) Extract, Certified Organic Rosmarinus Officinalis (rosemary) Leaf Extract, Certified Organic Salvia Officinalis (sage) Leaf Extract

First, we feel compelled to point out that this company is taking some liberties with the ingredient labeling laws, since aloe is the first ingredient, instead of water. This is a trick that many companies use because it makes their product look more concentrated because there's "no water." In reality, the water comes in from the Aloe Leaf juice, which is 99.5% water and only 0.5% solids based on industry standards. (Reference: Active Organics). But by including the water, they get to list it first on the ingredient list instead of at the bottom so it looks more appealing to potential consumers.

Based on the composition, we'd guess this product should stack up pretty well against a standard shampoo. It should clean your hair just fine, and the coco-glucoside should provide adequate lather. Most of the other ingredients will just rinse down the drain, though. And, if you're used to using a moisturizing shampoo that contain silicones or cationic polymers, you'll notice quite a difference in hair feel with this one.

What about styling? Creating a natural styling product is much more of a challenge, because styling products have to hold hair in place under a variety of environmental conditions. That's why hairsprays, gels, and mousses are made with hard holding polymers. Let's look at their own styling product, a gel.

Miessence Shape Hair Styling Gel Ingredients
Certified Organic Aloe Barbadensis (aloe vera) Leaf Juice, Certified Organic Ethanol (sugar cane alcohol), Organic Fermented Grain Extract, Certified Organic Rosa Rubiginosa (rosehip) Seed Oil, Chondrus Crispus (carageenan) Gum, Non-GMO Xanthan Gum, Certified Organic Pelargonium Graveolens (geranium) Essential Oil

The product descriptor contains the term "shape", and the website describes it as providing "medium body and hold for most hair types." Therefore, we think it's reasonable to expect this product to hold like a typical gel would. Unfortunately, a review of the ingredients does not reveal any fixative. This product certainly won't provide the kind of hold one you would get from a gel formulated with acrylate polymers (which most of the industry uses). The natural gums in this product will provide some style retention, but they don't have the humidity resistance or proper film forming properties to really hold hair in place. It would appear this would be much better positioned as a hair-conditioning leave-in treatment rather than a shaping product to provide medium hold.

THE BOTTOM LINE
Again, we stress that it's all about your expectations. If you would rather spend more money to ensure your products are free of "synthetics" and you're less concerned about matching the performance of "regular" products, then Miessence may be good deal for you. And bravo to Miessence for providing alternatives for consumers. However, they need to be careful not to imply that their products will function just as well as those with "evil" synthetic ingredients. While food grade cosmetics are a possibility, consumers need to be aware of potential trade-offs before spending a lot of money on them.

Will Brush on Block sunscreen protect my skin?

Betina would like to know…I saw an ad for a product called Brush on Block. It looks like a blush, but it works like a SPF 30 sunscreen. Is it too good to be true?

After looking into this product, we'd rate it "good" but not "too good."

A poorly applied sunscreen is worthless
Because of the potential for skin cancer, you really have to be careful when choosing the right delivery form for sunscreen. For example, even though there are a number of spray-on sunscreens on the market, the FDA has not yet approved sprays as a proven delivery vehicle, because more data is needed to show that they coat the skin evenly. In other words, even if the product contains the right active ingredients, you have to correctly apply them to skin or they won't work properly.

Powder is difficult to apply evenly
That's why Brush on Block (http://brushonblock.com/) concerns us: how do you make sure that a powdered sunscreen, which by definition consists of billions of tiny particles, cover your skin uniformly? If you apply this product like a regular blush or foundation you won't necessarily completely cover your face. If you miss even the tiniest of spots you could be opening yourself up for sun damage.

We're not the only ones with this concern. Even the Cosmetic Cop (http://thebeautybrains.com/DAOhb) (Paula Begoun, who sells powdered sunscreens) recommends not to use powder as your sole source of sun protection. Paula suggests, and we wholeheartedly agree, that you should use a sunscreen lotion and supplement it with a powdered sunscreen if you so choose. Layering different sunscreen products is a great way to make sure you're building up enough UV defense.

THE BOTTOM LINE

This product seems to be a great supplement to your daily lotion sunscreen, but to rely on it for your sole sun protection is dangerous, because you may not apply enough.

Do mole removing products work?

Barb asks...A salon in my town is offering a Groupon deal on a skin treatment called Rejuvi Spotaway. They advertise it as being able to remove brown spots and moles, and it is a topical product that is applied once in the salon. I'm interested but wary. Can anyone tell me if this is a good idea?

Moles are dark clumps of pigment that can become cancerous, and they should not be taken lightly! (pun intended.)

Mole misinformation
It's frightening how much bad information about mole removal products is out there on the inter webs. According to one astonishingly bad piece of information we found, if you want to avoid the expense and hassle of surgery, you can simply cut off the offending mole with a pair of scissors. Yikes! But when we went to debunk these mole minimizers, we were surprised at how hard it can be to find clear proof that something absurd is not true.

Trying to prove a negative
If we told you that sticking a green bean up your nose is an easy cure for a headache, you would be hard-pressed to find any evidence to the contrary in the scientific literature. No one would have wasted their time doing a study to disapprove such a ridiculous notion. You'd find plenty of information about what DOES work (especially when the subject deals with an over-the-counter drug) but you WON'T find a paper entitled "Results of a Double-blind Clinical Study Proving Nasal Injection of Phaseolus vulgaris (Green Beans) Resolves Cranial Pain." That's kind of how we felt when researching removal creams. There was no "smoking gun" that said mole removing creams were BS. So, we'll have to rely on a rather circumspect argument to make our case.

Reason 1: Mole removal creams are not legal drugs

First, there are no approved over-the-counter drug treatments to remove moles, that much was easy to establish. You can search for yourself by looking at the FDA's list of approved OTC monographs.

Reason 2: The mode of action is invalid

Some of the mole removing creams that we found supposedly work by using "acid" that caused the mole to dissolve. For example, here are the ingredients in the Spotway product that Barb asked: Deionized water, magnesium oxide, n-propanol, benzoic acid, triethanolamine, and phytic acid. We found other products which used "skin irritating" acids to "dissolve" the mole. This sounds suspiciously familiar to the type of salicylic acid products which ARE approved for removing warts. Okay, moles and warts are both skin bumps. Is it okay to use the same product for both? The answer is a resounding "Nope!" The Wart Remover monograph specifically says that this product should not be used on moles.

Reason 3: Medical professionals agree

We did find a well reasoned explanation of the whole issue on ZocDoc.com, but it wasn't credited to a specific medical professional, so we feel bad for including it. Still, it supports our point so here it is anyway:

Irritating the mole with a chemical cream will not make it go away. The only effective ways to remove moles are to have them surgically removed by a dermatologist or a cosmetic surgeon or, sometimes, to have them lightened up with the application of a laser based treatment. As always the diagnosis and the management of your particular skin concern will require a physical examination by your personal physician.

We also spoke to a couple of doctors off the record (hey, not everyone wants to have their name quoted on an anonymous beauty blog, go figure) and they both told us that based on their clinical experience, there is no safe and approved way to remove a mole by using a nonprescription cream. In fact, they were aghast at the notion of anyone attempting to remove moles themselves because moles can be pre-cancerous and need to be evaluated by a dermatologist. Melanoma is nothing to screw around with.

THE BOTTOM LINE

Unless this "mole removing" product is designed to kill vermin in your garden, you should have nothing to do with it. If you really are concerned about getting rid of pigmented patches of skin, please see a dermatologist first for your own safety.

How can body wash contain as many moisturizers as body cream?

Celeste says…I saw a bottle of Olay body wash that claims to contain as many moisturizers as a jar of Olay moisturizing cream. How is this possible?

You have to hand it to those rascals in the cosmetic industry. They keep coming up with claims that sound compelling but aren't really that meaningful.

First let's be clear about this: it is helpful to have moisturizers in body wash. Procter & Gamble, the makers of Olay, have some very nice technology that can disperse oily conditioners in a rich foaming system. But the idea that it's helpful to have a "jar full of Olay moisturizer's" in body wash is a little bit silly. Here's why:

How much moisturizer in skin cream?
The exact claim is "over a jar full of Olay moisturizers inside." We take that to mean that this bottle of body wash has (at least) as many moisturizers as a jar of Olay moisturizing cream. Looking the label of Olay's original Active Hydrating Cream, we see that the first moisturizing ingredient listed in the formula is petrolatum. Let's assume for the same of discussion that this formula contains 5% petrolatum. (It's probably somewhat less than that, but we'll use that number for a ball park calculation.) To find out the total amount of petrolatum in the Olay cream we just calculate 5% of 2 ounces to come up with 0.1 ounces.

How much moisturizer in body wash?
The Olay body wash is sold in a 23.6 ounce bottle. If you took the entire quantity of 0.1 ounces of petrolatum from the cream and put it in this bottle the formula would contain approximately 0.1/23.6 = 0.004% petrolatum. This is far too little to have any impact. The irony is that the body wash HAS TO contain far more petrolatum than that since it's the second ingredient in the formula!

THE BOTTOM LINE

This exercise isn't meant to imply that this body wash doesn't moisturize skin; we're sure it does. We're not even saying that the claim about the body wash containing more moisturizers than a jar of face cream is false; in fact it most certainly does contain more. We just think the comparison they're using is a bit silly because it doesn't mean anything.

What is micellar water?

Yvette asks...Lately I see a lot of brands coming out with something called micellar water. What are they, what do they do to skin? How are they different from regular water or a toner we all are used to seeing around? What do they put in there that makes it micellar?

Wow, we thought we'd seen it all when it came to Marketing co-opting technical terms to make products sound differentiated, but this is a new one! In reality, any product that contains a detergent (aka surfactant) can be called "micellar water."

What are micelles?
Micelles are the structures that surfactants form when they reach a certain concentration in water. Think of it this way: Surfactants are little chemical bridges with one end that loves water (hydrophilic) and one end that loves oil (lipophilic). When you dump a bunch of these molecules in water, the oil loving parts want to be close together to get away from the water. So, surfactant molecules spontaneously form these spherical blobs where the oily ends all point toward the middle of the sphere and the water loving ends all point to the outside of the sphere where the rest of the water is. That's why surfactants are so good at dispersing oil: oil droplets can "hide" from the water in the middle of the micelle so they can be suspended or washed away.

Once again, we point out that ANY product with surfactants will do this. It doesn't have to be called a fancy name like "micellar water."

Is there ANYTHING different about micellar water?
Here's a quick breakdown on the ingredients in these products. They typically contain the following:

• Water

• A Glycol (eg Hexylene Glycol, Pentylene Glycol) – acting both as a humectant and hydrotrope (improves solubility of the the makeup in the surfactant)

- Solubilizer (eg Polysorbate 20) – the surfactant that does the cleansing

• Preservative

• Fairy Dust

Based on the examples we've seen it looks like most of these products use non-ionic surfactants, which are very low foaming. So they're kind of like cleansers that don't feel like traditional cleansers. Non-ionic materials also tend to be milder than their anionic cousins, which include SLS, SLES, etc. So perhaps the "hook" for these products is that they look and act more like water than a traditional high-foaming cleanser.

THE BOTTOM LINE
If you're looking for a mild, low-foam face wash, micellar water may be just the thing for you. But don't be tricked into spending a ton of money just because of the micelles.

Is cuticle remover good for my face?

Kitten asks...Has anyone used cuticle remover on their face to get rid of dead, dry skin as in this Ezine article?

According to the article (http://thebeautybrains.com/nHy2r), getting rid of "dead, dry and all around ugly layers of your skin" is the first step to a brighter complexion. The article goes on to explain that cuticle removers are a "cheap and painless" way to remove dead skin. While we agree with the author that sloughing off dead skin is a way to brighten and smooth your complexion, we wholeheartedly disagree with the cuticle remover approach. Here's why.

Are cuticle removers safe for your face?

Most cuticle removers are based on chemistry that is similar to hair relaxers. That's because fingernail cuticles and hair are both made of keratin, which is a very tough protein. Keratin has a double bond structure (from disulfide bonds) which can only be broken down by aggressive chemical attack at a very high pH. Relaxers accomplish this with a variety of hydroxides (such as sodium, calcium, and lithium) in a cream with a pH of 13 or 14. (14 is the highest on the pH scale.) Here's an example showing that cuticle removers are also hydroxide based:

Nutra Nail's 30 second Cuticle remover Ingredients

Water, Glycerine, Potassium Hydroxide, Styrene Acrylates Co-polymer, Octoxynol 9, Sodium Dodecylbenzene Sulfonate, Carbomer, Stearic Acid, Aloe Vera (Aloe Barbadensis) Leaf Juice, Fragrance (Parfum)

Notice that potassium hydroxide is one of the first ingredients. Using our handy dandy litmus paper test strips we checked the pH and found it to be in the range of 13 to 14.

Applying high pH hydroxides to your face seems ill advised. If the hydroxide concentration is high enough, you could end up with skin burns. While this product is no doubt weaker than most relaxers, we would still be very concerned about leaving it in contact with the delicate skin of the face.

Are cuticle removers good exfoliators?

Okay, so the product is relatively cheap and potentially damaging to your skin. Does it provide some incredible benefits that offsets this danger? The answer is no. Skin doesn't have the same amino acid profile as hair and nails and therefore skin doesn't have the same kind of disulfide bonds to break. To remove the top layer of dead skin cells you need a chemical that reduces the adhesion of the cells so they slough off easily (without irritation). That chemical is salicylic acid, a beta hydroxy acid that can penetrate between the dead layers of your skin and loosen the scales. This product is on the acidic side (with a pH of around 3 or so), so some people may find it mildly irritating. However, it is much less likely to burn skin than a high pH solution of hydroxide.

THE BOTTOM LINE

Considering that there are safe and effective products that are NOT expensive, we don't know why anyone would try this potentially dangerous process. You should always be cautious about using cosmetics on parts of the body other than those it was specifically designed for.

Hair care questions

Do hair strengthening products really make hair stronger?

Tresemme was in trouble a while back because they made the claim that the product "makes hair 10X stronger after just one use". This proved too much for the Advertising Standards Authority (ASA), who is the regulatory body in the UK. According to the article we found, they received 3 complaints about the claim.

Making hair stronger
No shampoo or conditioner system actually makes hair stronger. If you do a test where you take the hair and pull it apart with an instrument like the Diastron, then measure the amount of force required to break the hair, you'll see no significant increase in strength. But this isn't how companies who claim hair strengthening support their claims.

What do hair strength claims really mean?
In response to the ASA complaints, Alberto-Culver said that stronger meant that it makes hair better-resistant to breakage and splitting. This is proven by using a robotic comb (a flogger) and counting the number of hairs that are broken after a given number of combing strokes. There is no doubt that they actually were able to support this claim. But this testing doesn't really prove that hair is made stronger. Shampoos & conditioners will not make hair stronger, at least none that are on the market today. The ASA agreed that this could be a method for supporting the claim, but they rejected the advertisement because they thought it was a little too misleading.

THE BOTTOM LINE
Understanding how cosmetic companies do their testing helps you be a smarter shopper, because you can choose to avoid companies that are making up their own definitions. (Although you won't have many left to choose since so many companies do this!)

Are sulfate free shampoos better for colored hair?

Tina's turmoil: I have been a longtime reader of another blog called Killer Strands and the writer (Dakota Ellis/Killer Chemist) is a hair colourist and a cosmetic chemist who has tested sulphate shampoos and proved it does fade color and may cause premature hair loss. She mentions it's very caustic when smelled and may cause you to to faint when opening a jar of SLS !

Sulfate shampoos do cause fading; however, they do not cause more fading than other types of shampoos. We can say that because we specifically evaluated all types of shampoos in unpublished research. But until that is published, it's just hearsay. If you really wanted to prove it to yourself, use 2 different shampoos on each side of your head the next time you get your color done. One should be a sulfate based shampoo and the other should be non-sulfate based. After 5-10 washes, you will not likely see any color difference between the two.

Dangerous sulfates?

The idea that sulfates make your hair fall out is just not true. No cosmetic chemist has ever proven this. Furthermore, while they are powerful degreasers and can dry out hair and skin, they are not caustic. And the notion that you will faint just by smelling a sulfate detergent is ridiculous. Sulfates have a weak, bland odor (it's true that inhaling concentrated SLS can irritate your nasal passages, but that will not make you faint.)

We have been in the cosmetic and personal care industry for many years and have not come across any published scientific study to show that sulfates are the worst thing for your hair color or would make your hair fall out. I suspect if you asked the Killer Strands folks for their data they won't have any. And without the data, it's just an unvalidated opinion.

Killer Strands

We looked up the Killer Strands website and it appears to be very professional and it contains a lot of good information. Dakota is doing a find job, but we couldn't find any references to specific studies backing up her statements. You need to consider that while Killer Strands does make some good points, they are also trying to sell you their products and services.

THE BOTTOM LINE

The Beauty Brains do not and will not sell cosmetic products. We do not recommend specific product brands and we encourage people to make up their own minds about what to buy. We present the unbiased science. If someone is trying to sell you a product, you have to read with skepticism everything that they write. It doesn't matter if they are cosmetic chemists, board certified colorists, or dermatologists. Once a piece of writing is put out there with the intent to convince you to buy a specific type of product, watch out. The information is suspect.

Is glycerin good for hair?

Cindy says...I always get confused about glycerin. Is it an ingredient I should use to combat my frizzy hair on hot, humid days? If so, how much can I add to my leave-in conditioner so it will be effective without being sticky?

Glycerin is what is known as a humectant. That means it has the ability to absorb moisture from the air and hold on to it. This is a very helpful property in skin lotions where it can help bind moisture to the skin. However, since humidity tends to increase the frizzing of hair, binding additional moisture is the last thing you want to do. I would stay away from glycerin in a leave-in conditioner to be used under high humidity. There is one possible exception: certain types of African American hair which are extremely dry may still benefit from glycerin even in high humidity.

Then why, you ask, do so many hair care products contain glycerin? Because it has a second property that is beneficial: It helps emulsions (like conditioners) maintain their consistency and keeps them from drying out.

THE BOTTOM LINE
Don't assume that all ingredients that are good for moisturizing skin are good for moisturizing hair.

Is this hair removal cream too good to be true?

Rita asks…A-Revitol hair removal crème says that it's so gentle you can use to remove pubic hair. I know that is a very delicate area so I am skeptical. Whats the deal?

The product in question is A-Revitol Hair Removal Cream. Here's the deal on the product claims and the likelihood that it will live up to those claims.

How do hair removal creams work?

All hair removal creams work essentially the same way: by using chemicals that dissolve the hair to a point where it can be wiped off. Since the hair is removed at (or just below) the surface of the skin, there's no razor stubble so your skin feels smoother than if you had shaved. Most products use a combination of two type of ingredients to dissolve hair: a thioglycolate and a hydroxide.

Is A-Revitol more gentle?

Any product potent enough to dissolve hair has the potential to irritate skin, but this product is formulated to be on the gentle side, because it only uses one of these two ingredients we just mentioned: a hydroxide (calcium hydroxide to be specific.) That means it's somewhat less likely to irritate skin, but it will also be somewhat less effective at removing hair.

A-Revitol Hair Removal Cream Ingredients

> *Water, Calcium Hydroxide, Mineral Oil, Petrolatum, Cetyl Alcohol, Stearyl Alcohol, Steareth-20, Peg-75 Lanolin, Glycerin, Aloe Vera Extract, Fragrance.*

Is A-Revitol a better product?

If you have really sensitive skin you might be better off with this product compared to a standard depilatory like Nair. However, since this product is almost 4 times the cost of Nair, you should probably try that one first to see if it works for you. (A-Revitol costs about $20 compared to $5 for Nair's Bikini Cream.)

Does the product do what it claims?

The key claim that the company makes is that it's safe enough to use anywhere, which is true enough as long as you follow their instructions to patch test it on your skin first. They are prone to some exaggeration, however. They say that A-Revitol will "get rid of hair in seconds" even though instructions tell you "leave the cream on for 12 to 15 minutes." "Instant" must be a relative term. The website mentions that "we sell countless numbers of these as we move toward a hairless society." If they're unable to count how many sales they make, they might want to fire their accounting department. And we must have missed the official announcement about the new hairless society.

THE BOTTOM LINE

A-Revitol appears to be a pretty standard hair removal product, but it might be right for you if you have really sensitive skin and you don't mind paying a lot more.

Do oils in shampoo really do anything?

Missy must know...I was looking for a good conditioning and found Garnier Triple Nutrition shampoo. Why is oil put in shampoo when its going to go down the drain because sulfates get rid of dirt and oil?

Garnier's Fructis line (made by L'Oreal) was originally based on fruit acids. Over time they've expanded their product line to include new products like this Triple Nutrition shampoo. According to their website, it's based on "Fortified Fruit Science", which consists of "3 Nutritive Fruit Weightless Oils": Olive, Avocado and Shea.

Fructis Triple Nutrition Shampoo Ingredients

> *Aqua/Water/Eau, Sodium Laureth Sulfate, Disodium Cocoamidopropionate, Sodium Chloride, Dimethicone, Glycerin, Glycol Distearate, Cocamide MIPA, Pyrus Malus Extract/Apple Fruit Extract, Parfum/Fragrance, Sodium Benzoate, Hexylene Glycol, Salicylic Acid, Guar Hydroxypropyltrimonium Chloride, Niacinamide, Pyridoxine HCl, Carbomer, Olea Europaea (Olive) Fruit Oil, Citric Acid, Saccharum Officinarum (Sugar Cane) Extract, Benzyl Alcohol, Persea Gratissima Oil, Persea Gratissima Oil/Avocado Oil, Linalool, Butyrospermum Parkii (Shea Butter), Ribes Nigrum (Black Currant) Seed Oil, Methyl Cocoate, Butylphenyl Methlyproprional, Sodium Cocoate, Citrus Medica Limonum (Lemon) Peel Extract, Yellow 5 (CI 19140), Camellia Sinensis (White Tea) Leaf Extract, Camellia Sinensis (Green Tea) Leaf Extract, CI 15985 (Yellow 6), F.I.L. D34974/2*

Nutritive Fruit Weightless Oils

As you can see from the ingredient list, these oils appear far down in the list, which means they're used at low levels. The main ingredients in the formula (the first 7 or so) are the ones that really get the job done when it comes to cleaning and nourishing (aka conditioning) your hair.

If you read their claims carefully, you'll see that for the most part they're very careful not to attribute functionality directly to the oils. The most explicit claim we could find was on Amazon.com, where they say this about the individual oils: "1. Olive oil - nourishes the inner core. 2. Avocado oil - nourishes and softens the middle layer. 3. Shea oil - nourishes and smooths the surface." Our guess is that they have some absorption data on these pure oils when applied directly to hair. But that's a far cry from what the oils will actually do when applied to hair from a rinse off shampoo at a very low level.

One more note: some oils (like silicone oils) can be formulated at high enough levels where they are deposited on the hair during rinsing. This kind of oil (at the right concentration) is an effective conditioning agent.

THE BOTTOM LINE

So why put in oils if they don't really work? The simple answer is "marketing." Every brand must have an interesting story to stand out, so just about every product has something that they tout as their "magic" ingredient. Good companies will carefully word the claims to only imply a connection; not so good companies will blatantly lie about what these featured ingredients can do. But almost everyone adds some "eye candy" to their ingredient list.

Is it okay to use fine hair products on thick hair?

Penny's plea...Is it okay to use fine hair products on thick/thicker hair? My hair isn't thick, but it isn't fine either, although it is more on the finer side. So is it okay to use fine hair products on thick(ish) hair, or should fine hair products only be used on fine hair and thick hair products only be used on thick hair?

Chemists do try to optimize products for hair types, but in many cases there really isn't that much difference. Here are the types of differences you might expect to see in products optimized for fine hair.

Fine hair versus thick hair
Shampoos

Formulators usually take one of two approaches when designing a shampoo for fine hair. One approach is to get the hair as clean as possible so as to not leave any residue that could weigh hair down. These formulations are essentially just gentle cleansers without any conditioners.

The other approach is to incorporate polymers into the shampoo that remain on the hair to give the fibers a little stiffness. This stiffness gives the hair more texture and makes it feel less fine and limp. These shampoos are cleansers combined with Polyquaternium-7, for example.

Conditioners

Conditioners for fine hair should avoid some of the heavier fatty conditioning agents like Behentrimonium chloride.

Styling products

In styling products for fine hair you may see some of the same polymer-based styling resins as holding agents, but used at reduced levels to avoid weighing the hair down.

THE BOTTOM LINE

In most cases there's not much difference between products for different hair types. But there's no harm in experimenting with fine hair products, because if you don't like them you can always wash them out.

How does this self-adjusting hairspray adjust?

Ronnie really wants to know...How can the hold of Philip B. Roth Self Adjusting Hairspray be adjusted? How does this work?

Wow. We don't mind products that use cleverly worded or intriguing claims to attract consumers attention. But this one is just plain ridiculous. How does the self adjusting product work? Here are the use directions straight from this website:

"For soft hold mist once

Medium mist 2 or 3 times

Firm hold mist 3 or 4 times."

Seriously? You adjust the hold by adjusting the amount you use??? There has to be more to it than that, doesn't there?

Nope. Looking at the ingredients we see this is a standard, water and alcohol based hairspray using ingredients that are available in many cheaper products. The two key ingredients that hold hair are the Butyl Ester of PVM/MA Copolymer and Octylacryla-mide/Acrylates/Butylaminoethyl/Methacrylate Copolymer. These exact same chemicals are available in products like CVS's aerosol Hair Shaping Spray, which is approximately 9 times less expensive.

Philip B. Roth Self Adjusting Hairspray Ingredients
SDA Alcohol 40B 190 Proof, Butyl Ester of PVM/MA Copolymer, Water (Deionized), Octylacrylamide/Acrylates/Butylamino-ethyl/Methacrylate Copolymer, Fragrance (Natural), Lauramide DEA, AMP, Benzophenone 4, Dl Panthenol, Phytantriol.

THE BOTTOM LINE
At $22 for 5 ounces, this is an outrageously over-priced product that doesn't "self adjust" better than any other hairspray on the market.

Do I have to use the same brand that my stylist tells me to use?

Sal says…I recently had a keratin hair straightening treatment. I was told to only use their products because they contain Juvexin, which was also in the original treatment. Is this a real ingredient or is it made up hype?

Juvexin is a combination of two Latin words: "Juv" from juven, which means youth, and "exin" from excise, as in cutting money out of your wallet.

Okay, we just made that up. Actually, Juvexin is a featured ingredient used in a line of products marketed by GKHair. The hair straightening salon treatments you referenced cost a few hundred dollars, according to what we saw on various websites. As with many professional products, it can be difficult to find an ingredient list online, so we can't say definitively what straightening technology this product uses. However, we did find a blog which claims the product is formaldehyde based. We don't know how your experience was, but this woman said the fumes from the product made her eyes tear up, which is very consistent with how formaldehyde systems behave.

What about Juvexin?

According to their website, Juvexin is their active ingredient, and it's "the ONLY protein compound which is scientifically proven to protect and restore hair back to its youthful state." Unfortunately, these claims appear a bit exaggerated (surprise!) as there are MANY protein compounds used to treat hair. (Unfortunately, without seeing the ingredient list, we can't tell which specific proteins are included.)

THE BOTTOM LINE

If you like these GKHair products and you can afford them, there's no reason not to use them. However, you shouldn't feel trapped into spending more on their "special" products just because of some Juvexin jive.

What do the oils in conditioner do?

Linda longs to learn…I've noticed that the Garnier Fructis Nutri-Repair Ultra-Nourishing Butter Mask has mineral oil fairly high up in its ingredient list, as well as olive oil and avocado oil further down in the list. The Nutri-Repair Conditioner has palm oil near the top of the list, and olive oil and avocado oil further in the list. Do these oils get deposited on our hair, and do they have any function in a hair treatment/conditioner?

Almost any kind of oil that helps lubricate to reduce frictional damage is good for hair. The trick is getting the oil on to the hair! Leave-in products do a really good job of this, because the oil is left in direct contact, but it's much trickier from rinse off products.

Suspended oils tend to rinse off

As anyone who's ever tried to make salad dressing knows, oil and water do not mix. That's why we use ingredients known as emulsifiers (also called surfactants) to help the oils disperse in water. But once these oils are emulsified, they tend to rinse away very easily, so they're just lost down the drain. There are some exceptions. Silicone oil, for example, can be delivered by a process called "dilution deposition." This is where the emulsion is designed to release the silicone when the conditioner is diluted, leaving the silicone to deposit on the hair. However, we've never seen this approach used successfully with vegetable or mineral oils because their chemistry is different. So, just because these oils are high on the ingredient list doesn't mean they are the main active ingredient.

So what makes Garnier conditioners work?

Look at the ingredients for both Garnier products (see below) and you'll see Behentrimonium Chloride and Stearamidopropyl Dimethyl-amine. These are the primary conditioning agents in these formulas. Also note the "methosulfate" ingredient. This is a mild quaternary ammonium compound that is able to stick to hair even after rinsing. It has a nice palm oil based fatty portion which gives the hair a nice slick feel. The formula also contains cetrimonium chloride which, even at low levels, will condition hair.

Do the oils do ANYTHING? Yes: they give the product a nice buttery feel during application. But that doesn't mean they actually stick around long enough to truly condition the hair.

Garnier Fructis Nutri-Repair Ultra-Nourishing Butter Mask

Aqua / Water, Cetearyl Alcohol, Paraffinum Liquidum / Mineral Oil, Dipalmitoylethyl Hydroxyethylmonium Methosulfate, Cetyl Esters, Ci 19140 / Yellow 5, Ci 15985 / Yellow 6, Niacinamide, Ribes Nigrum Oil / Black Currant Seed Oil, Saccharum Officinarum Extract / Sugar Cane Extract, Olea Europaea Oil / Olive Fruit Oil, Camellia Sinensis Extract / Camellia Sinensis Leaf Extract, Benzyl Alcohol, Linalool, Pyrus Malus Extract / Apple Fruit Extract, Pyridoxine Hcl, Persea Gratissima Oil / Avocado Oil, Cetrimonium Chloride, Methylparaben, Butyrospermum Parkii Butter / Shea Butter, Citric Acid, Butylphenyl Methylpropional, Citrus Medica Limonum Peel Extract / Lemon Peel Extract, Prunus Armeniaca Seed Powder / Apricot Seed Powder, Parfum / Fragrance

Garnier Nutri-Repair Conditioner

Aqua / Water, Cetearyl Alcohol, Elaeis Guineensis Oil / Palm Oil, Behentrimonium Chloride, Ci 19140 / Yellow 5, Ci 15985 / Yellow 6, Niacinamide, Saccharum Officinarum Extract / Sugar Cane Extract, Stearamidopropyl Dimethylamine, Olea Europaea Oil / Olive Fruit Oil, Chlorhexidine Dihydrochloride, Limonene, Camellia Sinensis Extract / Camellia Sinensis Leaf Extract, Linalool, Benzyl Salicylate, Isopropyl Alcohol, Pyrus Malus Extract / Apple Fruit Extract, Pyridoxine Hcl, Persea Gratissima Oil / Avocado Oil, Butyrospermum Parkii Butter / Shea Butter, Citric Acid, Butylphenyl Methylpropional, Citrus Medica Limonum Peel Extract / Lemon Peel Extract, Hexyl Cinnamal, Glycerin, Parfum / Fragrance

THE BOTTOM LINE

It's very common for companies to brag about the natural ingredients in their products to catch your attention. But you shouldn't assume that those ingredients are the ones that really make the product work.

Part 2: Scaremongering versus truly scary (Are cosmetics safe?)

If you believe everything you read on the internet you probably worried about lead in your lipstick, mercury in your mascara, and cancer from all kinds of cosmetics. Are beauty products really that dangerous? Is the industry really that uncontrolled? This chapter helps you understand why most cosmetics are safe to use and it warns you about the ones that really can cause you harm.

General questions

Why it's okay to have lead in lipstick

As you probably know, the subject of lead in lipstick has been a hot topic over the last few years. The age of the Internet has amplified the controversy and groups like the Campaign for Safe Cosmetics have added fuel to the fire by publishing papers and press releases scaring consumers about their cosmetics. It is enough to make you wonder...

"Why are companies allowed to put lead in lipstick?"

An excellent question that deserves an answer.

Lead Concerns

First, let's talk about why lead exposure is bad. Lead is a problematic ingredient because it can affect children's developing nerves and brains. Exposure can cause reduced IQ, slowed body growth, behavior problems and more. It is not as dangerous for adults but can still cause problems so exposure should be minimized.

Lead used to be very common in our environment as it was found in gasoline and house paint. It was added to these products for a number of reasons, but when scientists realized the harm being done regulations were enacted to stop the practice. Lead can still be found in some paints but much much lower levels.

Unfortunately, lead is ubiquitous and found naturally in everything including dirt, dust, water, soil, food, etc. You know those organic carrots that you are eating? They have lead in them. That ginger peach herbal tea? There's lead in there too. If you are a skilled enough chemist and have the right analytical equipment, you can find lead everywhere.

Lead in lipstick

Now back to our question, "why are companies allowed to put lead in lipstick?"

The simple answer is that they don't put lead in lipstick. It serves no purpose in cosmetics and is not used.

But you have no doubt read stories or otherwise heard about lead in lipstick and in other cosmetics. In fact, there is lead in lipsticks. As you may have figured out since lead is everywhere and in everything, there is going to be lead in lipstick. Some lipsticks have a higher concentration of lead because the naturally occuring red and pink colors have more more residual lead present.

FDA's stance on lead in lipstick
In the United States, the FDA is responsible for overseeing and regulating the cosmetic industry. The FDA doesn't set specific lead levels for lipstick but they do set levels for the colors used in lipstick. According to FDA rules, colors used in cosmetics may contain no more than 20ppm lead. The FDA says that the levels of lead in finished lipstick products are consistent with use of color additives that have allowable levels of lead. They also say that

"The lead levels we found are within the limits recommended by other public health authorities for lead in cosmetics, including lipstick."

Repeat study
There was, however, some debate over the data from previous tests that showed how much lead was in lipstick. So a new study (http://thebeautybrains.com/bL4dZ) was commissioned to test more brands (both in US and EU) using the FDA's validated method. Those results were published in the May/June 2012 issue of the Journal of Cosmetic Science. Here are a couple of interesting tidbits from the study:

• Average results from the study were very consistent with previous studies: on average lipsticks contain about 1 mg lead per kilogram of lipstick.

• While the study did not identify which companies manufactured the tested lipsticks, it did note that one brand in particular contained more lead than the others. (Even this brand was still within safe limits however.)

• The author found that certain shades contained more lead than others. Pink shades had the most lead followed by purple shades followed by red. The author theorized that the minerals used to lighten red shades may increase lead content.

The conclusion from the FDA is that the level of lead in lipstick is not a major health concern.

Should you be concerned?
We've established the fact that cosmetic companies do not add lead to lipsticks (or other cosmetics) and the the levels of naturally occurring lead found in these products are not a safety concern according to scientists at the FDA. But there is more about lead in lipstick.

One of the reasons that manufacturers do not remove naturally occurring lead from the colors used to make cosmetics is because it is chemically difficult to do. To separate lead from the mineral colors you have to use Hydrofluoric Acid. This is a strong acid that also has the effect of breaking down the color. So to remove residual lead, you often ruin the color.

The important part to note however, is that Hydrofluoric Acid is a much stronger acid than the ones found in your stomach and digestive system. If you did happen to swallow some lead-containing lipstick your body could not digest it. It just goes through your digestive system and gets excreted at the other end. The lead from lipstick is not absorbed in your body.

THE BOTTOM LINE
The levels of lead in lipstick are not harmful and this is not something you need to worry about. If you are concerned about lead in your

lipstick there is only one thing you can do, don't wear lipstick since every brand of lipstick contains some level of lead if you look hard enough.

Why lead in lipstick stories will never go away

This story about a study of lipstick (http://thebeautybrains.com/6OPrZ) done by the Daily Mail, which showed that 55% of lipsticks contained trace amounts of lead, leads us to conclude that this problem will never go away.

The problem?

No, not lead in lipstick. This isn't a problem. There is no credible study that demonstrates the level of lead in lipsticks is anything but safe. The problem is the belief that there is no safe level of lead or mercury or "toxin" that can be tolerated in cosmetics. Sadly, this is a problem that cosmetic chemists will have to deal with for the rest of time. Some people will never come to grips with the notion put forth by Paracelsus... (http://thebeautybrains.com/mgHo2)

> "All substances are poisons; there is none which is not a poison. The right dose differentiates a poison...." Paracelsus (1493-1541)

Why?

We've thought about this a lot, because it is such a frustrating topic for scientists. Here are five reasons we think this problem will never go away.

1. Fear stories are more compelling than safety stories.

This is just a truism of journalism. People are more interested in stories that scare them than in stories that are reassuring. Sensationalism sells. So stories of toxic cosmetics will always trump stories declaring cosmetics safe. And since cosmetics are far and away safer than most any other consumer product, the media will have to rehash stories about lead in lipstick. There just isn't much else.

2. People are scientifically illiterate

The reason that these fear stories are compelling is because people are generally scientifically illiterate. They also prefer simple answers to complicated questions. Lead = bad is a much easier thing for people to comprehend than "certain levels of lead are bad but other levels are perfectly safe". Scaremongering is effective because the people propagating the stories do so to a public that is not smart enough about science to make a judgment about the validity of the story. Did you know that, to determine the level of lead in lipstick, you have to use Hydrofluoric Acid to separate out the lead? The stomach acid just isn't strong enough to break down any ingested lipstick, so the lead will never get into your system anyway!

3. People are unable to properly evaluate risk.

Another huge problem is that people are just not good evaluating risks. They fret about lead in lipstick or BPA in plastic bottles, which have risk levels in the 1 in million lifetime risk, but think nothing of getting in a car which has a 1 in 100 lifetime risk of killing them. Here are the things that kill people (http://thebeautybrains.com/RoSGW). Cosmetics is not one of them.

4. Message benefits some marketers.

One of the reasons these stories will stay around is because some marketers use fear to set themselves apart from their competition. When you see "paraben-free" or "sulfate-free" claims on a container, there is the implicit claim that those things are dangerous or otherwise bad. These are not direct lies, but they implicitly propagate a myth and benefit from it.

Dunning Kruger effect.

Finally, there is the Dunning Kruger effect (http://the beautybrains.com/fyjJx). This is the notion that someone unskilled in a subject has more confidence in their opinion about the subject than someone who actually knows something about it. So, you get books written by PR agents and runway models exposing the toxicity & dangers of cosmetics. Why is it that people who have spent their careers researching and testing cosmetic products are not writing scare books about cosmetics? Why is it that the people who would most likely know the truth about whether cosmetics are dangerous don't pen these books?

Dunning Kruger.

THE BOTTOM LINE

Alas, this is the way of the world. Until we improve science education in our country and around the world, people are still going to find "Lead in Lipstick" stories compelling.

What's so terrible about propylene glycol?

Ally asks...I've been seeing "propylene glycol free" on a lot of products lately, together with 'paraben free' and 'mineral oil free'. Googled it to see what's so harmful about it and found the Material Safety Data Sheet, which warns users to avoid skin contact with propylene glycol, as this strong skin irritant can cause liver abnormalities and kidney damage.

Propylene Glycol (or PG as we cosmetic scientists call it) is primarily used in beauty products to improve freeze-thaw stabilize of emulsions. A few percent or less of PG can prevent a cream or lotion from developing a grainy, cottage cheese-like texture when exposed to low temperatures. It also has moisturizing properties similar to glycerine (which is more commonly used.)

But PG, along with many other chemicals, has gotten a bad rap from groups like the Environmental Working Group (EWG). For example, according to the website The Good Human the main role of PG is to "help any other chemicals that you come in contact with reach your bloodstream." and that it "alters the structure of the skin by allowing chemicals to penetrate deep beneath it while increasing their ability to reach the blood stream.

That sounds pretty bad, doesn't it? But let's take a look at what science really says about propylene glycol in cosmetics.

Why is propylene glycol used in cosmetics?
As we noted above the main reason for using PG in cosmetics is to improve product texture. Relatively small amounts, on the order of 2% or less, are required to achieve this effect. To be fair, we should also point out that PG is used at higher concentrations in a few products, where it acts as a solvent for other ingredients. But it is NOT primarily used to help other ingredients to penetrate into the blood stream.

Is propylene glycol dangerous in cosmetics?
According to the US Food & Drug Administration, propylene glycol is Generally Recognized As Safe (GRAS) for direct addition to food. It's also permitted for use as a defoaming agent in indirect food additives. The Cosmetic Ingredient Review board (a group of scientists who review the safety of cosmetic ingredients) have determined that it's "safe for use in cosmetic products when formulated to be non-irritating." Essentially this means that companies need to conduct skin irritation testing on new formulas to ensure PG doesn't cause irritation when mixed with other ingredients. This is a standard test that companies do on new products, so it's not a big deal. (By the way, the testing is done on people, not animals.) In addition, many oral and IV drugs use significant amounts of PG. It's our opinion that if an ingredient is safe for ingestion AND safe for use in injected drugs, it's unlikely to cause any problems in a topical cosmetic.

But what about skin penetration?
Let's be clear: propylene glycol is one of the ingredients that penetrates skin, but "absorption through the skin is minimal." Since PG itself is safe to ingest (it's either excreted in the urine or it breaks down in the blood to form lactic acid, which is naturally produced by your body), toxicity isn't really an issue. The only cases where PG getting into the blood stream caused a problem occurred when PG-containing creams where applied to large areas of burned skin. That makes sense, since burned skin would be missing the outer protective layer. In these cases, mild lactic acidosis and serum hyperosmolality were observed. There are certainly no problems when low levels of PG are applied to healthy, intact skin.

How much is PG is okay?
According to a report issued by the World Health Organization, the estimated acceptable daily intake for PG is about 25 mg of propylene glycol per kg body weight. (Seventeenth Report of the FAO/WHO Expert Committee, 1974). A 130 pound person would have to ingest about 3 pounds of PG per day before having any problems. And that's

by ingesting it; you could put MUCH more on your skin, since only a small amount actually penetrates through your skin into the blood stream.

What about penetration enhancement?

So PG is safe by itself, but what about helping other ingredients get through the skin? This is the one question we couldn't get a clear answer to. We couldn't find any studies showing which ingredients PG enhances penetration of and by how much. However, considering it's used in relatively high amounts in topical drug products, it seems unlikely to us that it will cause problems at the lower levels used in most cosmetics.

THE BOTTOM LINE

It's always good to be knowledgeable about the chemicals you put in or on your body. But based on the the most recent scientific data, it doesn't look like there's really much to be worried about from cosmetics that contain propylene glycol.

3 Reasons the EWG is a dubious resource

If you follow the cosmetic industry news, then you've probably heard about the Environmental Working Group (EWG) and their off-shoot group the Campaign for Safe Cosmetics. The EWG focuses on providing information while the CFSC attempts to get legislation passed. Ostensibly, they are consumer advocacy groups who endeavor to ensure that cosmetic manufacturers produce only safe products. That's a laudable goal, and one that we can all support.

However, cosmetic chemists, formulators and the cosmetic industry already support this goal, so the cosmetic products we produce are already safe. The EWG & CFSC are unnecessary. But we're certain that the good folks at these groups would disagree. From their perspective, cosmetics are not safe. And cosmetic chemists cannot be trusted to create safe formulas. They seem to believe that there are cosmetic chemists who want to create formulas that will poison their families and cause widespread cases of cancer. They don't think very much of cosmetic chemists or formulators.

Problems with these groups

The primary place that consumers (and beauty bloggers) find out about the EWG is through their online ingredient resource, called the Skin Deep database. It's an interesting concept, and they've clearly put a lot of work into it. Unfortunately, it is full of misleading information and many things that are just wrong.

Skin Deep database flaws

There are a few obvious flaws in the database that have been pointed out to the EWG, but they don't seem interested in changing them. Here is what we mean.

False information

There is false information in the database, but they don't seem interested in fixing it. For example, they have a listing for "Polyparaben." They even give it a chemical rating and call it an endocrine disruptor. Unfortunately, there is no chemical called "polyparaben". It doesn't exist. How they managed to come up with a toxicity score and links to studies about a non-existent chemical is baffling, and it certainly doesn't build faith in the reliability of their data. If they had a cosmetic chemist review the information they were putting up before entering it into the database, perhaps this wouldn't be a problem. Clearly, they don't. And they don't care to fix it, because this has been pointed out to them directly.

Nonsense ratings

Creating a hazard score is a dubious activity anyway (since it is the dose that makes the poison), but they aren't even consistent within their own scoring system. For example, they have listings for both Sodium Coceth Sulfate and Sodium Laureth Sulfate. Cosmetic chemists know that these compounds are essentially identical, with minimal differences. But somehow the Sodium Coceth Sulfate gets a 0 hazard score, while Sodium Laureth Sulfate gets a 4 hazard. This makes no sense.

Belief, not science

Perhaps the worst thing about the EWG Skin Deep database is that they are unwilling to modify their conclusions when new evidence comes to light. They base their actions on a belief and use science only when it supports what they want to believe. Since they are a politically motivated group, they are unable to accept new science which might indicate an ingredient is more safe than previously thought. There is not a single instance of them changing their stance on any cosmetic ingredient.

No courage of their convictions

But the most galling thing about the EWG is that they are hypocrites who either don't believe what they say or are more interested in making money off people than protecting them from "dangerous" products. For example, they list a Hall of Shame for sunscreens. In it they list specific products that are typical of "...what's wrong with the sun protection business." Of course, this does not stop them from making money through their Amazon Affiliate program by selling those same products. For example, they list Aveeno Baby Protection Sunblock as a Hall of Shame sunscreen because it is dangerous for babies, but they'll happily take your money if you want to buy the product. This means they either do not care that they are making money off of products that they believe are dangerous...or...they don't believe the products are really dangerous. Either way, it's shifty.

THE BOTTOM LINE
If the EWG & the CFSC is to be believed, cosmetic chemists are evil people who do not care about the safety of the formulas they create. We think this is BS.

Product recalls: how the cosmetic industry is kept safe

In the many years that we have spent formulating products, our companies never went through a recall. (A recall occurs when a company pulls their product off the store shelves in order to protect consumers.) We did have a microbial contamination issue with a pump imported from China that caused a big shipment of a new product to be scrapped, but it never made it to store shelves. This just demonstrates that cosmetic recalls are rare.

Or are they?

According to this story in Cosmeticsdesign.com (http://the beautybrains.com/0zgQg), there have been some significant recalls in the last year. And interestingly, they are for different reasons. Here are the ones they list.

Recent cosmetic product recalls

1. In the Banana Boat recall case people were catching on fire after using the product and then going near an open flame such as a grill. Turns out there was too much propellant and it didn't evaporate off the skin quickly enough. It would've been tough for the company to anticipate this problem. There is no standard test that would've caught it. We bet they'll develop one now, however.

2. Unilever had to recall their Suave Professionals Keratin Infusion Smoothing Kit because of a record number of complaints.

3. J&J recalled some Aveeno baby care lotion after the FDA found that it was contaminated with too much bacteria. (Tell us again why it is a good idea to remove proven preservatives in favor of unproven ones?)

THE BOTTOM LINE

Recalls in the cosmetic industry are pretty rare, which is a tribute to the effectiveness of current regulations. (You should see how many food products are recalled each year.)

Despite what you've been told, cosmetics ARE regulated

Consumer advocacy groups frequently claim that the cosmetic industry is unregulated. This is false. The regulatory framework for the cosmetic industry was set up in 1938 with the passage of the Food, Drug and Cosmetic Act. This created the FDA, who regulate the cosmetic industry.

You can find more about the FDA cosmetic regulations here. (http://thebeautybrains.com/8Gty1)

Perhaps what they really mean is that the FDA is not strict enough with their regulation of the cosmetic industry. This is a reasonable claim, but how can you judge whether or not this is true? We're of the opinion that you have to look at the results of the current regulatory system to determine whether it is effective. And since the cosmetic industry has an excellent record of safety, it would be difficult to claim that things need to become more strict. If they did become more strict, how would you measure whether the products are safer? How unsafe are they right now? How many less injuries would be reported? Without a baseline to prove the current level of safety, it makes no sense to make more regulations.

Incidentally, the FDA has recently been cracking down on cosmeceutical type claims that are being made by the big cosmetic companies. Both Avon and L'Oreal have been sent warning letters (http://thebeautybrains.com/JQaet) about some of their anti-aging cosmetics.

THE BOTTOM LINE
Unregulated? We don't think so.

Is It safe to transfer cosmetics to another bottle?

Bebe says...Often, by the time a skin care product or makeup item has reached its expiration date, I still have a lot left. I'm thinking of putting a portion of such products in another bottle when I open it, and giving that to a friend. Are there any products that I shouldn't do that with? I wonder about antioxidants which break down when exposed to oxygen.

You should be able to transfer most products, provided you follow a few simple rules.

Guidelines for transferring cosmetics
1. Use a clean, dry bottle to reduce the chances of bacterial contamination

2. Use a bottle of similar material. For example, don't transfer perfume from a glass bottle to a plastic one, because the solvents in the fragrance may cause the plastic to crack.

3. Only transfer small amounts of products that are light or oxygen sensitive and fill the container as much as possible. Leaving as little headspace as possible will help prevent oxidation.

THE BOTTOM LINE
You can safely transfer cosmetics to different packaging. However, that doesn't mean you can transfer ANY cosmetic to ANY package. Use a little common sense and you should be fine.

Cosmetic companies shouldn't cave to fearmongers

Recently, Johnson and Johnson have announced plans to remove a variety of chemicals (http://thebeautybrains.com/arsXI) from their cosmetic products. This is strictly a PR move, and also an unfortunate mistake for the following three reasons.

1. Emotion trumps science

From a cosmetic chemist standpoint, the ingredients we use are safe. Even J&J admits that the formulas that they are currently selling are safe. But despite the guaranteed safety of their product, they are going to change them (http://thebeautybrains.com/xW6LI)...

"Because we know parents want complete peace of mind when making decisions about their babies, we will phase out the use of all parabens from our baby care products."

So in other words, they don't really care what the toxicologists, independent scientists, and government regulations say; if parents are irrationally afraid of parabens, they are going to remove them.

We suppose it's not that big of a deal at the moment. But how about when the next fearmonger group comes out and convinces a tiny minority of consumers that surfactants are dangerous? Is J&J going to remove all surfactants from their products? Or thickening agents, or pH adjusters, or any other ingredient that people are irrationally afraid of? Good luck with that.

2. Alternatives may be less safe

The one piece that fearmonger groups miss is that when a cosmetic formulator has to switch from a material with a proven safety profile, they replace it with something that is less tested. J&J might be phasing out perfectly fine ingredients like Quaternium-15 and Methylparaben, but what will they be switching to? A brand new preservative that has only a few years of safety testing? Do you know the long-term exposure effects of the material? Not likely. They could easily be using materials that are less safe than the current options. Congratulations, CFSC. You just made everyone less safe.

3. Encourages scientific illiteracy

The third problem we have with this move by J&J is that they are encouraging scientific illiteracy. They are capitulating to non-scientific thinking and rewarding willful ignorance. This is the same kind of nonsense that will prompt people with no background in climate science to declare that global warming isn't happening or that vaccines are causing autism. These are the non-scientific, irrational positions that are having a real, detrimental effect on our government and society. J&J is contributing to the erosion of society. Nice going.

Chemical free cosmetics

Perhaps the dumbest thing we've seen related to this issue are the various tweets and blog posts declaring that Johnson and Johnson are removing chemicals from their products (http://thebeautybrains.com /W4M6Y). How J&J goes about making "chemical free" cosmetics is a mystery to us. Last time we checked everything that goes into their cosmetics is a chemical.

THE BOTTOM LINE

As scientists, we have a real problem with capitulating to non-science based conclusions about chemicals. If an ingredient is unsafe, then by all means get rid of it. But if it is safe, publicly reformulating is a mistake. We understand cosmetic companies have to give consumers what they want, and that's what J&J is doing. It just doesn't feel right to give in to irrationality.

The problem with avoiding chemicals

We've read a few articles about what people called the "toxic trio" in nail polish and it really bugged us.

Toxic nail polish

The basic premise of these articles is that most nail polishes contain toxic ingredients that make them dangerous, and that consumers should choose polishes that do not contain these ingredients. In one, the author goes through and points out some studies that supposedly support her point. They don't. Here are a few examples:

"DBP can irritate your stomach, eyes, and upper respiratory system." - It's not surprising that a volatile compound can be irritating, but this is true of many compounds and doesn't make nail polish toxic.

"phthalates found in mothers can be particularly harmful, causing reproductive damage to sons." – I don't know what this has to do with nail polish. Are women drinking nail polish? Where is the research showing phthalates from nail polish are getting through the nail and into the body?

Then the author talks about Toluene and says in low doses it is safe. So why talk about high doses?

Finally the author propagates common fears about formaldehyde, despite the fact that the levels used in nail polish are not harmful.

Uncertain alternatives

But what really bugs us is the advice to try a brand that doesn't have the "toxic trio". The problem is that the author is quick to conclude that nail polish containing the toxic trio are unsafe, but doesn't even investigate the chemicals in the products that she recommends. The nail polish brand that she recommends is not more safe than other nail polishes.

All one has to do is look at the safety profiles of the alternative chemicals in the recommended brand. As alternatives to Toluene, this manufacturer uses Butyl Acetate. According to the MSDS for Butyl Acetate, "The substance is irritating to the eyes and the respiratory tract. The substance may cause effects on the central nervous system. Exposure far above the OEL could cause lowering of consciousness."

And the carcinogen potential of Butyl Acetate (http://the beautybrains.com/yX89G) has also been investigated, and they concluded that "TBAc (butyl acetate) should be considered to pose a potential cancer risk to humans because of the metabolic conversion to TBA."

This is somehow safer?

THE BOTTOM LINE
There is little evidence that the "toxic trio" or "toxic trio-free" nail polishes are unsafe. They are safe. It just bugs us to see myths like these propagated.

Are you confused about alcohol in cosmetics?

Sharky says: I am a little confused re: the use of alcohol in skincare products; can anyone help me with which ones are not good for the skin and which ones are beneficial? Also, what does it mean when a product range is certified halal?

There are two kinds of alcohol used in cosmetics that can be drying to skin:

Alcohol in cosmetics
• Ethyl alcohol (also listed as Ethanol, Alcohol Denat or SD Alcohol)

• Isopropyl alcohol (also listed as isopropanol).

These are drying to skin because they are short chain alcohols (very few carbon atoms in their backbone), which means they are liquids and can act as solvents. They can dissolve the natural protective oils in your skin.

Other kinds of alcohols can actually be good for your skin, because they are long chain fatty alcohols, which means they act like an oily moisturizer. The most common ones include:

• Cetyl Alcohol

• Stearyl Alcohol.

Halal cosmetics
Essentially, "halal" means the product is lawful according to The Islamic Food and Nutrition Council. In the case of foods, you must avoid the following:

• Pork and pork by-products.

• Improper slaughter techniques for animals.

• Ingredients made from carnivorous animals.

• Intoxicants like alcohol.

You can learn more about halal products here:
http://www.ifanca.org/halal/

THE BOTTOM LINE
Just because a cosmetic contains alcohol doesn't mean it will be drying to your skin.

Cosmetic ingredients that can be harmful

There is so much ridiculous scaremongering about the dangers of cosmetic ingredients that people often ignore cosmetic ingredients that can actually be harmful. Here is a list of cosmetics and cosmetic ingredients that can be dangerous. Now, this doesn't mean consumers can't use them and that you can't formulate with them; it just means you need to be careful and label your products properly.

Relaxers
One of the most dangerous types of cosmetic is a hair relaxer. This product uses Sodium Hydroxide or other high pH bases that can cause severe burns on the scalp if left on for too long. You need to be extremely careful when using a product like this. It's something that is probably best left up to professionals.

Perms
Here's another hair treatment that can be dangerous. Perms use thioglycolates to cause a chemical reaction that rearranges the chemical bonds within hair to help create the curl. This chemical can cause burning and be sensitizing if left on the skin for too long.

Depilatories
These products are great for removing hair, but they can also cause significant irritation, especially if the product is misused by the consumer. Patch testing should be required before using to ensure that there will be no significant allergic reaction. Thioglycolates are also used to make this product work.

Hair color
The thing about hair products that makes them more dangerous than skin products is that the hair is "dead" tissue. Strands of hair are no more alive than shoelaces. Therefore, chemically reactive ingredients can be used (if done carefully). Hair color is another type of reactive chemical that is used as a cosmetic. While it can be used safely, it can also cause problems if used incorrectly. The reaction can irritate or burn skin, and the ingredients can also have a severe reaction to your

eyes. This is why there is a warning not to use hair coloring on your eyebrows.

Skin bleaching agents

While not technically cosmetics, skin bleaches are often sold as such, and they can be dangerous if used improperly. The primary concern is skin irritation.

Sunless tanners

This ingredient isn't dangerous per se, but it can cause your skin to turn orange, and most consumers would not want to experience that. The ingredient, DHA, chemically reacts with skin protein to cause the orangish/brownish color and if not used properly, uneven, undesirable colors can result.

THE BOTTOM LINE

For the most part, cosmetic products are perfectly safe to use. The scaremongering about cancer, toxicity, and hormone disruption is unproven and in contrast with what the majority of professional toxicologists believe.

Cosmetic industry and chemical scaremongering

We received the following press release from the Public Relations people at Pantene. As beauty bloggers, we get lots of these things and we mostly ignore them (unless they pique our interest for some reason).

This one from Pantene caught our eye with this headline:

> "Get Frizz Free – Without Formaldehyde! Achieve Pantene Pro-V hair without the harsh effects."

The press release recounts the dangers of using formaldehyde containing hair straighteners (like Brazilian Blowout), asking:

> "With dangerously high levels of formaldehyde linked to illness in hair stylists and their customers, are you willing to risk your health for smooth hair?!"

This warning is followed with a pitch for their solution:

> "Luckily, you won't have to put your health in jeopardy to achieve frizz-free locks if you use the Pantene Pro-V Restore Beautiful Lengths Frizz Control Shampoo and Conditioner and Restore Beautiful Lengths Smoothing Balm!"

Chemical scaremongering

The thing that bugs us most about this press release is that they call-out a specific ingredient and focus on how dangerous it is to your health. This is exactly the kind of chemical scaremongering that groups like EWG and Campaign for Safe Cosmetics rely upon to manipulate a misinformed public.

Indeed, the FDA did warn the Brazilian blow-out people that their product is improperly labeled. But when Pantene makes the further claim that...

> "With dangerously high levels of formaldehyde linked to illness in hair stylists and their customers, are you and your readers willing to risk your health for smooth hair?!"

...they are just playing into people's fears and possibly lying. The Brazilian Blowout is not linked to illness in customers. It has not even been linked to illness in stylists, but rather it has been demonstrated to exceed limits for health and safety. This represents a danger to stylists, not consumers, as this press release says. Then when they say

"...you won't have to put your health in jeopardy..."

if you use Pantene, they are just selling a product based on fear, not based on superior performance. This is exactly the kind of junk marketing that natural and organic players use when they bash Pantene and other mass market brands.

It's really a terrible way to promote a product. It makes people fearful and chemically ignorant.

Market your benefits
Now, we're in agreement with the FDA that the Brazilian Blowout product should be reformulated or removed from the market, but we think it is wrong for Pantene to use the incident as a way to market their own product. They are just propagating the scaremongering marketing that so frequently harms their own brand.

THE BOTTOM LINE
If the Pantene product is useful for anti-frizz, then that is what they should advertise. It should not be implied that it's a safer way to straighten hair (which it won't do.)

Parabens: a tale of two headlines

There was a recent study on parabens that made the news. It was research published in the Journal of Applied Toxicology conducted by Dr. Philippa Darbre and Mr Lester Barr.

The key findings of the research includes:

1. Parabens were detected in 99% of all breast tissue samples

2. An average of 85.5 ng/g was found. Four times higher than work done in 2004.

3. Propylparaben and methylparaben had the highest levels detected

The researchers conclude...

Mr Lester Barr – "Our study appears to confirm the view that there is no simple cause and effect relationship between parabens in underarm products and breast cancer."

Dr Darbre – "The fact that parabens were detected in the majority of the breast tissue samples cannot be taken to imply that they actually caused breast cancer in the 40 women studied."

Darbre further concludes that the fact that parabens are found in breast tissue justifies further investigation.

What's the story?

The study is interesting and presents a bit of a mystery. Why are parabens being found in breast tissue? Where are they coming from? As Darbre says, more research is needed.

But the story we most want to write about is the way that this story is being reported.

Take a look at these different headlines about the same press release.

From Science Daily...

> "Parabens in Breast Tissue Not Limited to Women Who Have Used Underarm Products"

From Cosmetics Design...

> "Study finds no link between deodorant use and breast cancer"

Then from Red Orbit...

> "Possible Link Between Personal Care Products, Breast Cancer Studied"

And NHS...

> "Deodorant chemical 'found in breast tumours'"

And finally Healthcareglobal.com

> "Popular cosmetic chemical found in breast cancer tissue"

Viva la difference

How is it that all of these media outlets got the same press release and came up with completely different headlines?

None of these headlines are lies per se. But they all communicate a different message. The Science Daily headline (which we view as the least biased source) captures what we see as the main point of the study. Parabens are found in breast tissue whether people have used deodorants or not.

The Cosmetic Design headline is clearly biased to tell the story in a way that exonerates the cosmetic industry. They don't lie, but they do miss the point of the research.

The next few headlines are much more sensational, however, and communicate the message that the study somehow links parabens, cancer and the use of cosmetics.

The study does the exact opposite!! It just goes to show that way you tell a story is just as important as the facts that go into creating it.

THE BOTTOM LINE

In our view, this research provides no new information to the debate. Unfortunately, chemophobes will look at this research as a new reason to ban parabens from cosmetic products. *Sigh.*

Cosmetics and cancer

As scientists, we're concerned about how the Campaign for Safe Cosmetics and the Environmental Working Group are using scaremongering to scare consumers away from beauty products that are perfectly safe to use.

Competitive Enterprise Institute

We're excited to see that the Competitive Enterprise Institute is now committed to exposing the facts behind the propaganda that these groups are spreading. According to Dana Joel Gattuso, author of the CEI Issue Analysis, The True Story of Cosmetics: Exposing the Risks of the Smear Campaign:

> "As part of their effort to ban the use of synthetic ingredients from skin products, environmental extremist groups are working to incite fear among consumers, making outrageous and bogus claims that we are poisoning ourselves by using lipstick, makeup, deodorants, skin creams, and even baby products."

These groups claim certain preservatives cause cancer, create neurological disorders, or cause hormone disruption, while in fact, when used properly, these ingredients protect users from bacteria that can cause eye infections, skin rashes, and even deadly infections such as E. coli and Salmonella. Similarly, the EWG claims the sunscreen ingredient, oxybenzone, can cause skin cancer, even though cancer research organizations such as the Skin Cancer Foundation refute this claim.

Pending legislation

Perhaps the most disturbing point is that these groups are lobbying for the Safe Cosmetics Act of 2011, which would "ban any cosmetic and skin care ingredients that exceed a one in a million risk of an adverse health impact. That bill would effectively ban most ingredients since almost everything carries risk greater than one in a million." CEI's tongue-in-cheek video makes the point nicely.

Skin care/makeup questions

Will drying your nail polish with UV lights give you finger cancer?

Ruby asks…How likely is it that you will get skin cancer from gel nails? Would putting sunblock on your fingers before getting a gel mani help?

Given the legitimate concerns raised about UV tanning beds causing skin cancer, it seems perfectly reasonable to be worried about similar health dangers from the UV lights used to cure gel nail polish. (The UV radiation causes the polymers in the polish to "cross-link", which makes the polish harder and longer lasting.)

When we first heard about this, we speculated that using sunscreen would protect your skin around the nail bed but that the nail polish itself should absorb UV radiation, so it wouldn't pass through your nail to the skin beneath it. But now we have data that definitively answers this question. (At least as definitive as you can get from a single study.)

Are UV nail lamps safe?

According to an article by Heather Onorati, which was published in the December 12, 2012 edition of Dermatology Times, researchers from three hospitals (Massachusetts General Hospital, Boston, Alpert Medical School of Brown University, and the Veterans Affairs Medical Center, Providence, R.I) measured the UV light produced by these nail drying lamps. They compared their output to the FDA's guidelines for photo devices that have already been proven to be safe. Results showed that the nail drying lamps produce only a "tiny fraction" of these other devices and therefore they "do not appear to increase the lifetime risk of skin cancer."

THE BOTTOM LINE

Based on the best science to date, nail drying lamps do not pose a significant cancer risk. So it looks like gel nails are safe after all!

Does your Vitamin C lotion contain a dangerous ingredient?

Elen asks…I've recently heard that sodium benzoate when met with ascorbic acid (vitamin C) can lead to cancer and damage DNA. Is it true?

The concern stems from the fact that sodium benzoate can release benzene, which is a chemical that has been linked to cancer.

Why is sodium benzoate in my cosmetics, and can it really form benzene?

Sodium benzoate is a preservative that helps protect your creams and lotions from micro-organisms. This story has it roots back in 2005 or so, when trace amounts of benzene were discovered in a variety of soft drinks. Benzene is found in a variety of petrochemical products (like emissions from burning coal and oil, gasoline service stations, and motor vehicle exhaust) and in cigarette smoke. In this case the benzene was apparently being generated by the decarboxylation of the benzoate by ascorbic acid. This was of concern, because benzene has been linked to several types of cancer.

The FDA investigated and found that most of the soft drinks had less benzene than is allowed in water. (The FDA sets limits for water, but not other beverages.) The limit for water is 10 parts per billion (ppb). (Remember we're all exposed to chemicals that, at low levels, are perfectly safe – the dose makes the poison, as they say.) The soft drink manufacturers that were exceeding the 10ppb decided to reformulate their products, and those have now dropped to much lower levels. So for now, there doesn't appear to be any concern for soft drinks. But what about cosmetics?

Definitive data is needed

Vitamin C lotions certainly can contain sodium benzoate. But since no one's published data, we don't know if these cosmetics undergo the same reaction that occurs in beverages. Since we know that sugar inhibits the creation of benzene, it's possible that similar ingredients in cosmetics (like sorbitol) could have the same effect.

Since no one has done a definitive study on cosmetics (that we're aware of) we don't know what the benzene levels are. (Perhaps individual manufacturers have tested some of their own products. If they have, it would be nice if they would share that data.) It's difficult to guess, but it seems doubtful there's much to worry about. We know that the pH has to be below 2 for benzene formation to occur and not many cosmetic products are in that ranges. Even if small amounts are formed, there's less risk to you than if you were ingesting the same amount (because it won't all penetrate your skin.)

THE BOTTOM LINE
Okay, lots of info here, but what to do? It looks like even under the worst conditions (with the highest level of benzene directly ingested into your body), the risk of cancer is still low compared to environmental exposure to this chemical. If you don't find that reassuring enough, then we see only one other option. Your only choice for true peace of mind is to avoid Vitamin C products that contain sodium or other benzoates. Fortunately, this is easy enough to do by reading the ingredient list.

What is kajal and is it safe around my eyes?

Rachel asks...Is Himalaya Herbals Kajal safe to put around eyes? What ingredient gives it pigment?

Before we can talk about this specific product, we need to explain what is kajal is.

Curious about kajal
Those of you not familiar with kajal may recognize it by its more common name: kohl, which is a pigment that has been used since ancient time in parts of Asia and Africa to darken the area around the eyes. ("Kajal" typically refers to kohl eyeliner while "surma" refers to kohl powder.)

Historically, kohl was made from a sulfide of lead which, as we all know now, is not the safest of chemicals to expose yourself too. While some old-school kohl/kajal products still exist, most modern versions (like STILA Kajal Eye Liner) use the name, but not the lead. Instead, they use iron oxide pigments (like those used in mascaras), which are much safer and give the same basic effect.

Is Himalaya Herbals kajal safe?
Here is where it gets tricky. Unfortunately this company, like many others, does not provide full ingredients lists for its products online. All we've been able to find is what they refer to as the "key ingredients", which to us is just marketing speak for "we're only going to tell you about the ingredients we want you to know about." Still, for the sake of completeness, here are the ingredients that we were able to find:

> *Almond Oil (Prunus amygdalus, Vatada) Camphor (Cinnamomum camphora, Karpura) Castor Oil (Ricinus communi, Eranda) Rose (Rosa damascene, Shatapatri) Triphala consisting of the fruits Emblica officinalis (Amalaki), Terminalia chebula (Haritaki) and Terminalia bellerica (Vibhitaki)*

It's obvious that this formula must have more ingredients, since there's nothing here that contains a black pigment. It's likely that the product uses an iron oxide just like most other companies do you. But, since in their infinite wisdom they've chosen not to share that information with us, there is no way to know for sure that they are not using a lead compound.

THE BOTTOM LINE
Unless you can get the company to provide a full ingredient list, we would err on the side of safety and buy a product that's honest and open about the ingredients it contains.

Is nail polish safe?

Patty asks...Something I've been curious about lately is the risk of toluene in Seche Vite top coat, and I was wondering if you could elaborate on it...At what concentrations/volumes does toluene become toxic? Could the amount in SV be dangerous? Is it true toluene cannot be absorbed through the skin, as it is non-polar?

Here's the scoop on toluene:

1. Most of the data on toluene has been conducted on inhalation exposure, as this had been the major exposure route. (It was used extensively as a solvent in the printing industry for many years). Authorities in most countries around the world have set an atmospheric concentration of 100ppm. This limit is based on very long exposures in the work place. Safety limits are set by finding the highest level at which no effect is seen and then applying a safety factor to this.

2. If the product is not used correctly or abused, there certainly could be enough in there to present a hazard. Don't go around sniffing the stuff.

3. Toluene can be absorbed through the skin, but very very slowly. Absorption through the nails would be even lower, probably negligible.

THE BOTTOM LINE
If you use this product occasionally and use it in a well ventilated area, it appears unlikely that it poses much of a health hazard. If you're are constantly exposed to high concentrations of its fumes, that's a different story.

Can I make my own aluminum free deodorant?

Gabby asks...After reading your blog post about scare tactics, I decided to try my hand at homemade deodorant. I looked at all kinds of recipes, and I created one based on the available ingredients I had in my kitchen. The result was amazing! I was so excited to have created a natural, "aluminum-free" deodorant that worked. Then, I researched a little more and realized that the clays I was using have aluminum content. I went back online and noticed that many natural deodorants contain clays that have aluminum. Can you help me figure out if it can be called aluminum-free if it contains bentonite clay, for example? Also, how does this type of aluminum fit into the neurotoxicity issue?

First a little background about the different kinds of aluminum in Antiperspirant/Deodorant products.

How is Aluminum used in antiperspirants?
Ingredients: Aluminum zirconium tetrachorohydrex glycine

Function: These ingredients are designed to interact with the pores of your body, creating tiny gelatinous plugs that reduce sweating. The best research to date shows no connection to Alzheimer's disease.

How is Aluminum used in deodorants?
Ingredients: Bentonite, Kaolinite

Function: These are naturally occurring clays that are used as thickeners because of their ability to gel/thicken the solvents typically used in deodorants. We have not been able to find any reference linking these to the Alzheimer's controversy.

Can you legally claim aluminum-free?
Unfortunately, we're not lawyers (although we do like to watch them on TV), so we can't really advise you of the legality of making such a claim. You're certainly free to make such a product for your personal use, but if you plan on selling your own deodorants, we recommend consulting an attorney.

THE BOTTOM LINE
Regardless of what legal council tells you, would this claim really pass the "red faced test" for you? In other words, if you really don't believe the scientific consensus that says aluminum salts in APs are safe, then can you in good conscience add aluminum containing ingredients to your deodorant? If science says they're safe, they should be safe in both cases.

Can Retin-A kill you?

Belinda is bothered...Given that retinoids are so good at building collagen, thickening the dermis and making skin texture better, I'd like to use it on my legs (entire circumference of the thighs) to help improve the texture of thinning, slack, "crepey" skin. I'm worried, though, about absorption into the bloodstream, as I've heard that retinoids used in large amounts can cause vitamin A toxicity. I realize that Tazorac is a synthetic retinoid, but don't know whether that means it bears no resemblance whatsoever to Vitamin A, or whether it's simply a synthetic form of the vitamin? And even if it's not, then could large-scale application of Tazorac still be dangerous?

We're cosmetic scientists, not toxicologists, but we did find two interesting references that might help answer your question. And just for the record, Tazorac is a brand name for the drug tazarotene, which is a retinoid (http://thebeautybrains.com/HYz5j) product related to Vitamin A.

Is Retin-A toxic?
According to the first reference, a study from PubMed (Journal Med Toxicol. 2009 Jun;5(2):73-5), (http://thebeautybrains.com/kcsBj) a massive acute overdose of Retin-A (aka Tretinoin) doesn't seem to present much of a problem. In an suicide attempt, a 31 year old man ingested 1000 mg of Retin-A, which is about 100 times the normal dose. The only apparent negative side effect he experienced was diarrhea. So it looks like the body can tolerate a high, one time dose of Retin-A, and there's no way you'd ever absorb that much through your skin! But what about a lower dose over a prolonged period of time?

The second reference (Medscape) (http://thebeautybrains.com /mpMdx) is chockfull of info on retinoids, and it states that very little (up to 6%) of the retinoids you apply to your skin end up in your blood stream. This was based on a study showing that "levels of retinoic acid in the blood are not increased by twice-daily application of 0.025% tretinoin to more than 40% of the body surface area over a 1-month period." That comment is as close to a definitive answer as we could find.

THE BOTTOM LINE

Based on the studies we found, it seems unlikely that rubbing a Retin-A type product all over your body will kill you. Regardless of what these studies say, however, you should still check with your doctor before using retinoids (or ANY drug) in a way that's inconsistent with its directions. And remember, there is another danger besides toxicity: pregnant women are warned about using retinoids because of their potential teratogenic effect on fetuses.

Is citric acid bad for skin?

AA asks...A cleanser I'm using contains citric acid, and although it is lowish on the ingredients list, I'm not sure that it's low enough to just be in there for adjusting the pH. The website says that their products are gentle enough to use straight after cosmetic procedures such as chemical peels and laser resurfacing, but then why add citric acid, which would surely lead to scarring in these situations?

Here's the ingredient list for the product in question:

> Water, Sodium Cocoyl Isethionate, Stearic Acid, Glycerin, Aloe Barbadensis Leaf Juice, Stearyl Alcohol, Disodium Cocoamphodiaceate, Sodium PCA, Phenoxyethanol, Caprylyl Glycol, Hydroxyproply Methylcellulose, Coco Glucoside, Glyceryl Oleate, Allantoin, Glycyrrhiza Glabra (Licorice) Root Extract, Citric Acid, Disodium EDTA, Chrysanthemum Parthenium (Feverfew) Extract, Camellia Sinensis Leaf Extract

It appears that the citric acid is placed at the right spot on the ingredient list, and we doubt it's present at a very high level. Remember that (in the US) ingredients are listed in descending order until you get to ingredients that are present at less than 1%. After that you can list them in any order. In this product we'd say the 1% line is about where glycerin is, so anything after glycerin can be listed in any order.

Also, the primary surfactant, Sodium Cocoyl Isethionate, is one of the mildest that money can buy, so this product does appear to be properly formulated for the uses that you described.

THE BOTTOM LINE
Unless your dermatologist tells you otherwise, this product appears to be safe for use after chemical peels and laser resurfacing. (Assuming, of course, you're waiting a reasonable amount of time after the procedure before washing your face.)

Why does my doctor tell me NOT to wear nail polish?

Nadia needs to know... I'm having sinus surgery on my nose, but my doctor said to be sure not to wear nail polish during surgery. I can't figure out what nail polish on my fingers has to do with an operation on my nose. I'm too embarrassed to ask my doctor. Can you explain it for me?

Nadia, we're cosmetic scientists, not medical professionals, but we can guess why your doctor is concerned about your nail polish.

Love is like oxygen

During surgery, doctors track vital signs like your heart rate, blood pressure, and the amount of oxygen in your blood. Blood oxygenation is measured using a little device that clamps on to your finger which is known as a "pulse oximeter." The oximeter works by shining light through your finger nail and measuring how much light is absorbed. The more light that is absorbed, the more oxygen that is in your blood. Your doctor could be worried that nail polish could interfere with this measurement. But is this concern valid?

Interestingly, the answer may be "no." A study (http://the beautybrains.com/DPDGA) conducted at the University of Southern California has shown that nail polish does NOT interfere with the pulse oximetry. The study revealed that neither nail polish nor artificial nails significantly interfered with light absorption from the device.

Say "no" to nail polish

So, does that mean you can ignore your doctor's advice and where a nice shade of OPI to your sinus surgery? I'm afraid not! There's another reason that wearing nail polish in the operating room is a bad idea. Surgeons have a "backup" way to check blood oxygen just in case the pulse oximeter fails. It's called "looking at your nails." If your blood oxygen drops to a dangerously low level, your fingernails will start to turn blue. Nail polish will mask this color change, so the doctor won't be able to visually check your blood oxygen. The risk is very low, but by keeping your nails unpolished, you're helping your doctor keep you safe.

THE BOTTOM LINE
Beautiful nails are not worth the risk! Even though the odds of anything going wrong in your surgery are very small, you should still listen to your doctor's advice and NOT wear nail polish the day of your procedure.

Is sunblock giving my baby cancer?

Princess is perturbed...I've been using Aveeno Baby Sunblock Lotion on my 2 year old, but I read that it contains dioxane, which causes cancer. Should I switch sunscreens?

Dioxane is a contaminant that is linked to cancer. However, there's little reason to be concerned about it in your cosmetics.

What is dioxane?
The chemical you're referring to is actually 1,4-dioxane. It's not an ingredient, so it won't be listed on the package, but it is a contaminant that shows up in small amounts in some cosmetic raw materials. Typically it comes from ingredients that have "PEG," or "Polyethylene" in the name. In the case of the Aveno sunscreen it comes from PEG-100 stearate, which is used to dissolve the oil soluble ingredients in the product.

Can this chemical be dangerous?
Yes, under some conditions. 1,4 dioxane was linked to cancer in animal feeding studies done in the 1970s by the National Cancer Institute. Given that danger, the FDA decided to conduct additional studies to determine if the chemical can penetrate skin when applied from cosmetics. They found that yes, it can. But they also found out that since the levels of 1,4 dioxane in cosmetics are low and that since it evaporates relatively quickly, very little actually gets into the skin. So this appears to be another case of an ingredient that is carcinogenic at very high levels but does not pose a danger under normal use conditions.

THE BOTTOM LINE
Is sunblock safe? Yes, according to the FDA: "The 1,4-dioxane levels we have seen in our monitoring of cosmetics do not present a hazard to consumers." Furthermore, they say that their testing shows that levels of 1,4 dioxane are actually decreasing due to improved manufacturing processes. For more details, including full technical

references, see the FDA's report on 1,4 dioxane. That's good enough for us.

Is mouthwash poisoning our water supply?

Janice asks...When I was in 6th grade, my teacher claimed that Listerine (remember this was the 1980s when it was still amber colored and tasted like medicine) was poisoning our water table. To this day I wondered how much truth was in what she claimed. She said that when we spat the Listerine into the sink it would work its way into the water table and we'd end up drinking polluted water.

This claim does have the ring of an urban legend about it, so we checked Snopes.com to debunk it but had no luck. So, we'll have to do this the hard way. Let's see if we can find any evidence that Listerine is poisoning the water supply.

Listerine ingredients
There are four key active ingredients that make Listerine so, uh..."Listeriney." (The rest is pretty much water, alcohol, flavor, color, etc.)

• Eucalyptol (0.092%)

• Menthol (0.042%)

• Methyl Salicylate (0.060%)

• Thymol (0.064%)

We did a little research on each of these to determine a) how toxic they are and b) how likely they are to build up in the water supply.

Eucalyptol
Eucalyptol oil can be poisonous if you chug down enough. Based on the medical record, it looks like you'd have to swallow about half an ounce before you'd have serious symptoms. Even then, among people who ingested that much, almost all recovered within a day or two. Plus, consider that you'd have to swallow about 2 dozen bottles of Listerine to get half an ounce of pure Eucalyptol. Furthermore, having Eucalyptol diluted in water makes it even more difficult to ingest enough to be a problem. Is swallowing small amounts over a

long period of time dangerous? We couldn't find any direct data, but it's not soluble in water, so it is easily separated out during purification processes. (http://thebeautybrains.com/WRnkF)

Thymol

This ingredient has been well researched and found to degrade rapidly in water (DT50 16 days.) Therefore, the risk of environmental pollution is low.

Reference: D. Hu and J. Coats, Evaluation of the environmental fate of thymol and phenethyl propionate in the laboratory, Pest Manag Sci 64:775–779 (2008)DOI: 10.1002/ps.1555

Menthol

Menthol is taken orally in a number of forms including candy (as part of peppermint oil) or cough drops. The typical human oral dose is 60-120 mg menthol, so this won't be poisonous even at high levels in the water supply (http://www.inchem.org/documents/jecfa/jecmono /v042je04.htm, http://thebeautybrains.com/bfUh9)

Methyl Salicylate

If we've said it once, we've said it 5 or 6 times: the dose makes the poison. Methyl salicylate is used in small amounts as a flavoring agent at no more than 0.04%, but at high concentrations or in its pure form, it is toxic. The lowest published lethal dose is 101 mg/kg body weight in adult humans. You many have also heard the story of the seventeen-year-old cross-country runner who died in April 2007 from topical absorption of methyl salicylate from muscle-pain relief products. Luckily, the potential for bioaccumulation is low, because although methyl salicylate is soluble in water, it is readily biodegradable, so it will not be persistent.(http://thebeautybrains.com/itCec, http://thebeautybrains.com/JHqZZ/, http://thebeautybrains.com/a7TDu)

Fun Bonus Fact

Listerine is named after Joseph Lister, one of the fathers of antiseptic surgery. If he had lent his first name to this product instead of his last, it would be called "Josephine" and that would be just plain weird.

THE BOTTOM LINE

While we don't pretend to be toxicologists, based on the information we've found, there doesn't appear to be much credence to the notion that Listerine is poisoning our water supply. Of course, we're sure all the Listerine Deniers will beg to differ.

Is teeth whitening bad for enamel?

SB says...I've always had white teeth until I got my braces. My teeth have become yellowish with huge black spots after I removed my braces. Is there is any way to whiten my teeth without thinning my enamel? (Using strawberry to rub on the teeth is a bad idea according to my dentist, as it contains acid.)

We have to admit that we've never heard of whitening teeth by rubbing them with a strawberry, but then again we've never been much for fruit-based beauty solutions. We have, however, heard that whitening teeth can harm enamel. Is that true or is it just another beauty myth?

Dental myths
According to Dr. Alexandre Gause of Smile Design Manhattan (a dental professional and fan of the Beauty Brains), this myth is busted. Dr Gause says the effects of whitening agents on tooth structure have been studied and have been found to have no negative effects of the integrity or hardness of teeth. He cited a study which showed that microhardness of enamel and the underlying dentin of teeth whit- ened with an in-office system, the strongest of any whitening agents, were statistically equivalent to those only brushed with toothpaste or rinsed with only water!

THE BOTTOM LINE
Based on the latest research, teeth whitening processes do NOT weaken tooth enamel. Next: we find out if a strawberry daiquiri has a beneficial effect on teeth (or anything else)!

Shaving dye danger

As regular readers of the Beauty Brains know, we urge you to be skeptical when it comes to scaremongering about cosmetic ingredients. In too many cases, people claim cosmetic ingredients are dangerous, when the best science available says they're safe. But we also try to present a balanced perspective, so when real safety concerns are raised we want to bring those to your attention as well. Case in point, a recent study shows that some dyes used in cosmetic products may present a danger when used on freshly shaved skin (http://thebeautybrains.com/tCGzH).

Danger from dye?
The study focused on two blue dyes that have been used in food and cosmetics, Brilliant Blue and Patent Blue V. While the dyes did not penetrate normal healthy skin, they were found to significantly permeate shaven skin. (Because the concern is specifically related to shaved skin, the article mainly focused on men's aftershave products, but we assume the same risks apply to shaving legs and, ahem, other things.) This discovery raised concerns because of health risks associated with systemic absorption of these kinds of dyes, because these dyes have been associated with allergic reactions, particularly for asthma prone individuals

Should you be concerned?
The opposing point of view, from the International Association of Color Manufacturers (IACM), questions the validity of study. The IACM says the report is "misleading" and "unnecessarily alarming," because these ingredients have been safely used for over 90 years. Given the long period of time that these dyes have been safely used, and considering that they are only likely to affect some people, the risk doesn't seem to be high.

THE BOTTOM LINE
While the risk is very low, it appears that more research is needed to confirm the results of this study to ensure these dyes remain safe for

use. If you are prone to allergic reactions, you could screen your cosmetics to avoid these dyes. (Which won't be easy because FD&C Blue 1 is widely used. Patent Blue V is less of a problem because we couldn't find any reference to Patent Blue V (aka Food Blue 5) being used in cosmetics in the U.S.) Check the ingredient list for these Color Index numbers: CI 42090 and CI 42051.

Is it safe to mix sunscreen and insect repellent?

Jenny's just concerned... I was told that products that are combination sunscreens and insect repellents may not be safe. Is this true?

Malicious mixing

According to an Associated Press report, there have been a few small scale studies (done on animals and human skin cells, by the way) that indicate mixing sunscreen actives with DEET (the insect repellent active ingredient) might not only increase skin penetration of DEET, but also reduce efficacy of the sunscreen.

The FDA put out a notice asking for comments to determine if this is a problem or not. The PCPC (Personal Care Products Council) says that the small studies that showed the problem are flawed. So what happens next? More research.

Certainly this is an important issue that merits further research, but there may be a more immediate reason for concern. Think about how these products are designed to be used: Sunscreens need to be repeatedly applied, in fairly large quantities, to keep your skin covered. But insect repellents are only intended to be applied occasionally (to prevent over exposure).

THE BOTTOM LINE

A combination sunscreen/insect repellant may sound like a great idea, but the two kind of cancel each other out in a weird way — if you apply enough product to give good sun protection, then you might be overdosing on the insect repellent. But if you lower the dose of the repellant, you don't get enough sunscreen. Thank you very much, but we'll just carry two separate products in our beach bag.

Is Octocrylene a safe sunscreen?

Lisa asks...Why is Octocrylene being targeted as being dangerous? I am hearing all kinds of conflicting info about chemical sunblocks.

Hmmm, this sounds like another scaremongering story, but let's dig a little deeper to find out if this controversy is really fact or just another beauty myth.

Crying over Octocrylene
To begin, it's helpful to understand why we need Octocrylene in the first place. Does it do anything different from all the other sunscreens we have? The answer is yes: it provides improved sun protection. Although by itself Octocrylene isn't a very good sunscreen, it can protect other UV absorbers from breaking down, and it can even boost their performance. It also helps them coat the skin better. So Octocrylene is a great tool for boosting sunscreen efficacy.

As with all sunscreens, it has been thoroughly tested before it was approved. In the US, Octocrylene has been evaluated by the FDA and is considered safe for use of up to 10% in the formula. Similarly, the EU allows its use up to 10% in a formula while Health Canada allows a maximum use level of 12%. With three independent approvals, this looks pretty safe, so why the controversy? There are two reasons.

Potential irritant
There are a number of reports in the literature about Octocrylene causing irritation. Octocrylene had 2 reported cases of irritation in 2003, but according to an article published in the Contact Dermatitis journal, reports of positive patch testing have been increasing. Here's some additional information from Medscape about sunscreen allergies. The Archives of Dermatology and the Dermatology Journal Online also discuss allergic responses to Octocrylene.

One theory is that Octocrylene appears to be a strong allergen, leading to contact dermatitis in children and mostly photoallergic contact dermatitis in adults with an often-associated history of photoallergy from ketoprofen (a pain reliever). Patients with photoallergy from ketoprofen frequently have positive photopatch test reactions to octocrylene. These patients need to be informed of sunscreen products not containing octocrylene, benzophenone-3, or fragrances.

DNA damage?

The second part of the controversy is more serious, because it involves potential DNA damage. Octocrylene is one of those ingredients that can be absorbed into the skin, and some studies have shown that it may promote generation of potentially harmful free radicals when exposed to light. Since free radicals can damage DNA, there is concern that this ingredient might have contributed to an increased incidence of melanoma in sunscreen-users compared to non-users. Researchers say further studies are warranted to determine the true health impact of this ingredient.

THE BOTTOM LINE

This beauty myth does have a kernel of truth to it. It seems like there is some legitimate concern regarding irritation for children and some adults, so some (still a minority of the population) will want to avoid it. And further research is warranted into the free radical damage that this ingredient could potentially cause.

Why Is sodium lauryl sulfate in my night cream?

Grace asks…Why sodium lauryl sulfate is in my night cream designed for face? I do understand why they put it in shampoos, shower gels or face cleansers. But why on earth would they use it in a cream intended for staying on my face all night long? I am kind of freaking about it now.

Sodium Lauryl Sulfate (SLS for short) is a high foaming anionic surfactant and is most often used in cleansing products, like you mentioned above. However, it may be found in creams and lotions, because it also used as part of emulsifying waxes or polymer suspensions. At low levels like that, there's probably no reason to freak out.

However, given that SLS can be irritating (especially when left in contact with the skin) and that there are a a wide range of other emulsifiers available, there's really no need for this ingredient in a cream. If you ask us (which you did), that's just sloppy formulating. We recommend finding another night cream.

THE BOTTOM LINE
Even though sodium lauryl sulfate is safe when used properly, it just doesn't make sense to include it in a leave in product. Looks like it's time for a trip to Sephora for you.

Is it safe to use an expired acne product?

Erica asks... Due to pregnancy and breastfeeding, I stopped using my AcneFree Severe set with main component BP 2.5/ 10%. Now I noticed the date on them is March 2012. Can these still be used? And if yes, for how long?

If you were asking about a cosmetic product, we'd say that if the product is only a couple of months out of date and there are no apparent signs of deterioration (in other words it looks and smells okay), it's probably fine to use for another few months at least.

Drugs are different

However, in this case you're talking about a drug product. And the active ingredient in this acne product (Benzoyl Peroxide) is very temperature sensitive and degrades rapidly at any temperature much above room temperature. The main decomposition product of benzoyl peroxide is benzoic acid which will not have the same effect on your acne.

THE BOTTOM LINE

There's really no point using a product if it's not going to be effective, so you should replace it.

The media Is scaring people away from sunscreen

Articles like this bug us.

"The Claim: A Sunscreen Chemical Can Have Toxic Side Effects" (http://thebeautybrains.com/QDUWs)

In this sound-bite, headline reading world, a person will casually see this in their reader or on the Internet and conclude that sunscreens are toxic. The fact is further supported in the first paragraph, where the writer says, "Sunscreen is supposed to protect skin. But some people suspect that a chemical in sunscreen, absorbed through the skin, may be even more hazardous than the sun's rays."

The author then goes on to cite a couple of small studies that some people find supports the headline. But if you read a little further down the article, you see a completely different story.

According to the independent researchers at Memorial Sloan-Ketterin Cancer Center, the research raising toxic concerns of Oxybenzone are unrealistic, and oxybenzone is safe for use at normal levels. They also looked at the data for the compound being tested on humans and found there were no safety concerns.

THE BOTTOM LINE
We appreciate the fact that they end with the bottom line that "exposure to oxybenzone, through normal sunscreen use, is safe..." but what's with the "sunscreeens are toxic" spin?

Ridiculous.

Hair care questions

Are keratin hair straightening products safe?

Mandy must know...Brazilian Blowouts were found to release formaldehyde. Are the Keratin-based hair-straightening products that I see stylists in salons doing that much safer on hair/environment?

The safety concerns regarding high levels formaldehyde in hair straightening products have been well documented, and inhaling large quantities of formaldehyde gas is a legitimate health concern. (see http://thebeautybrains.com/MLJyb) Some of the Brazilian Blowout type products contained as much as 10% formaldehyde, which far exceeds the safe limits. (Remember: the dose makes the poison!)

The Keratin straightening products you refer to use an entirely different chemistry. They typically contain cysteamine, which also reacts with the protein structure of your hair, but is safer from a health perspective than the classic Brazilian Straighteners. However, it also doesn't straighten as well. And, because it chemically reacts with protein, it can damage and weaken your hair to some extent. (Much less damage than using a relaxer but more than simply combing and brushing.) However, this chemical does NOT raise the same health/environmental concerns as high levels of formaldehyde.

THE BOTTOM LINE
Keratin hair straighteners are safe and effective, although they won't tame your hair as well as formaldehyde-containing products or relaxers will.

Does baby shampoo contain eye numbing ingredients?

Sahar says...I think this is an old urban legend that has been going around for years.

People keep saying that Johnson & Johnson 'No more tears' baby shampoo contains secret numbing agents so that a baby's eyes won't sting if the shampoo gets in them. I think that any numbing agent would be required to be listed in the ingredients label. They keep insisting that numbing agents are in there, despite all evidence to the contrary. Can you settle this once and for all? Is there anything in J&J baby shampoos that would numb a baby's eyes?

Don't worry, Sahar, there are no numbing agents in the J&J's baby shampoos.

J&J No More Tears Baby Shampoo Ingredients

> *Water, Cocamidopropyl Betaine, PEG 80 Sorbitan Laurate, Sodium Trideceth Sulfate, PEG 150 Distearate, Fragrance, Polyquaternium 10, Tetrasodium EDTA, Quaternium 15, Citric Acid, Yellow 10, Orange 4, Sodium Hydroxide (may contain).*

How baby shampoo works

One of the key attributes in producing a no-more-tears formula is the micelle size (micelles are aggregations of surfactant molecules); the bigger they are the less irritating they are. The theory is the bigger micelles cannot penetrate the eye membrane and hence cause irritation. The pH of the product, salt content, and impurities in the raw materials are also critical.

When we first heard this urban legend, the "numbing" properties were attributed to the ingredient benzyl alcohol. I believe it was part of the preservative system in J&J baby shampoo at one point in time, but it's no longer used in this product. It is, however, still contained in a few of J&J's baby lotions.

THE BOTTOM LINE

Baby shampoos are less irritating, because they leave out ingredients that can sting your eyes. They don't add in anything to mask the irritation.

Can men's hair dye take the color out of my skin?

Ally says...Watch out folks. Started using Just For Men hair dye last summer – once per month, and developed vitilligo. JFM co. is paying for dermatologist treatments etc, so they know there is a problem. Their box now warns about vitilligo. I don't believe it did back when I started using it last summer. I could be wrong about that, but clearly they know about a connection now.

When we saw AFL's comment we were immediately skeptical. We expected the reason the company is paying his doctor's bills is that it was cheaper than going to court. So we searched the literature for a connection between this product and vitilligo, but we didn't really expect to find anything. Hoo boy were we wrong!

The hair dye – vitilligo connection
Until we checked it out, we didn't realize that JFM contains para-phenylenediamine (PPD), a chemical used in hair dyes that is known to cause sensitizing problems in some cases. In particular, PPD is known to cause skin depigmentation in some individuals. (The chemical affects the melanocytes which produce skin color.) Whether or not this is exactly the same condition as vitilligo we can't say, but the end result is the same: white patches on your skin that may or may not ever resume their natural color. As AFL pointed out, Just For Men includes the following warning statement on their package:

"In rare cases, use of hair dye has been associated with skin depigmentation (skin lightening or loss of skin color), which may be temporary or permanent. If you notice any skin depigmentation or other allergic reaction such as discomfort or severe itching, discontinue use immediately.

Do not use this product at all if you have depigmentation problems such as white patches on your skin (a condition called vitilligo) or if you have a family history of skin depig-mentation problems, as an allergic reaction may cause temporary or permanent loss of skin pigment."

Just For Men Hair Color Ingredients

Water, Coco Glucoside, Amino Methyl Propanol, Carbomer, Isopropyl Alcohol, Fragrance, Isopropyl Acetate, Trisodium EDTA, Erythorbic Acid, 2 Methyl 5 Hydroxyethylaminophenol, 1,2,4 Trihydroxybenzene, P Phenylenediamine, Sodium Sulfate, P Aminophenol, N,n Bis (2 Hydroxyethyl) P Phenylenediamine Sulfate, Sulfuric Acid, Cinnamidopropyl Trimethyl Ammonium Chloride

THE BOTTOM LINE

While there is cause for concern, you shouldn't freak out about this. MANY people use this product (and other hair dyes that contain PPD) without any problem. But for those individuals who are susceptible to this condition, PPD can cause a real problem. Always do a patch test as recommended by the manufacturer and discontinue using the product if you have any issues.

Are organic shampoos safer?

Bernice begs to know... I was looking at claims of several organic cosmetic brands, and one Suki blew my mind. There are so many "harmful" ingredients listed that they needed two pages... Is the situation that bad with regular cosmetics containing synthetics? Okay, I could understand the issue with triclosan, but what about cocamidopropyl betaine (which, funny enough, is used as a primary surfactant in many other organic brands) or let's say, lanolin? Should we be that paranoid?

Bernice, we salute your skepticism!

Beware of misinformation
There's so much wrongness with the information in Suki's list that it's hard to know where to start debunking it. They're not even consistent with their warnings – cocamidopropyl betaine is bad because "it contains a significant petroleum component..." but their own shampoo contains shea butteramidopropyl betaine, which contains the same petroleum component. While we're looking at the shampoo, on their list to avoid is denatured alcohol, but ingredient number 2 on the ingredient list is SDA Alcohol, which is not just a similar chemical - it is the same chemical.

Also, lanolin certainly used to contain a lot of pesticides, but with pesticide usage more controlled and improvements to the refining process, the level of pesticide residues in cosmetic and pharmaceutical grade lanolin these days is lower than required for foods. We could go on...sigh.

THE BOTTOM LINE
The information provided by Suki is proof that you can't believe everything you read on the internet. We're sure they make wonderful products, but you shouldn't be scared into spending more than you need to on "organic" cosmetics that aren't really any safer.

Why is sodium hydroxide in my conditioner?

Fanny is furious...Why is sodium hydroxide in my Herbal Essences conditioner? Will it take my hair out? YIKES!!!

You can rest easy, Fanny. Herbal Essences won't cause you to lose any hair (unless you're pulling your hair out after trying to figure out all their overly cutesy names.)

Sodium hydroxide is safe
After looking at a few Herbal Essences conditioners, we noticed that only some of them, such as Hello Hydration, contain NaOH (that's chemist talk for sodium hydroxide.) Here are the ingredients:

> *Water, Stearyl Alcohol, Behentrimonium Chloride, Cetyl Alcohol, Bis Aminopropyl Dimethicone, Orchis Mascula Flower Extract, Zea Mays (Corn) Silk Extract, Cocos Nucifera (Coconut) Fruit Extract, Fragrance, Benzyl Alcohol, Disodium EDTA, Sodium Hydroxide, Methylchloroisothiazolinone, Methylisothiazolinone, Blue 1*

We're not sure why some versions use it while others don't, but in any case, it's there for one reason: to adjust pH. While NaOH is damaging to hair when used at high concentrations and at high pH, when used at low levels at neutral pH, it doesn't cause any problem at all. That's because sodium hydroxide is basic (high pH) and it will react with other ingredients that are acidic (low pH). This reaction neutralizes the hydroxide so it's not harmful to hair.

THE BOTTOM LINE
While you should always be on the look out for "suspicious" chemicals in your personal care products, you also have to understand that the concentration of the ingredient and the form that it's used in have a large impact on how dangerous the ingredient really is.

Part 3: Makeup or Make Believe (Popular Beauty Myths)

Remember that scene in the movie "My Big Fat Greek Wedding" where Gus says to use Windex to get rid of zits? Everyone has heard one of these "old wives tales," or urban legends, about some special beauty treatment. Sometimes these crazy ideas really work and sometimes they just make you look silly. This chapter helps you separate fact from fiction when it comes to home beauty remedies.

Skin care/makeup questions

Does my skin breakout because it's getting used to a new product?

Mary asks...I've heard people comment that they used X product (skin cream, miracle serum, etc.), and that it caused breakouts for the first week or so, as their skin purged itself of toxins, but was thereafter a wonderful product. This sounds like bunk to me—if a product is good for your skin, wouldn't it be good from the first day? Are these breakouts really the skin purging itself of toxins? I always thought a breakout was a breakout—indicating something not good for the skin. When I use a product (moisturizer, etc.) and it causes a breakout, I stop using it—have I been too hasty? Should I give it another chance?

This is a tricky question, because it's such an entrenched and beloved interpretation of what sometimes happens as your skin adjusts to a new skin care regimen. While we agree with your assessment that this "sounds like bunk", we decided to check with one of our dermatologist friends to find out for sure. Here's what the doctor had to say:

First, here's the bad news for those who believe that your skin breaks out because it's getting rid of toxins: there is no scientific basis for this "toxin purging" concept in skin care. Skin pores, oil glands, and sweat glands are complex structures, but the harboring of, and purging of, toxins just isn't something we have a lot of evidence for them doing. That said, I won't ever claim that scientists have any story all figured out. So, while we can't help you understand a 'break out' as a toxin purge, we can provide a more grounded explanation for it: It's called "perifollicular inflammation" which means redness and swelling around the pore.

It's known that using a product that is keratolytic (dead skin cell and blackhead busting) will allow comedones (big plugs of dead skin, sebum and stuff stuck in your pores) to loosen. When this debris becomes lose it can 'rattle about' in the pore causing inflammation and ultimately a pimple-like bump. Eventually this plug of skin debris will pass out of your pore leaving it blessedly unclogged. This process explains why an acne product such as Retin A (tretinoin) can 'make acne worse before it gets better'. So, this 'purging' of comedones may explain the 'toxin purging' myth that you inquired about, comedones being 'toxic' to look at and always unwanted. But, and this is the big but, it could also be that the new product is actually worsening acne.

THE BOTTOM LINE

So there you have it – another beauty myth busted! Acne products can make your skin look worse before it gets better, but it's not because of any "toxins" being released from your skin. It's because of the biology of comedone formation.

Your skin lotion can set off airport explosive detectors

According to this article on No More Dirty Looks (http://thebeautybrains.com/YaWLV),certain brands of skin lotion can be read as explosives by Airport detectors. Sounds like an urban legend, doesn't it? Let's take a look....

Do cosmetics contain "explosive" ingredients?
Cosmetics themselves are not explosive. If they were, we'd have warehouses of cosmetics blowing up all the time. But ammonium nitrate, the fertilizer used to make illicit explosives, is used in a few cosmetics as a buffering agent.

Is there enough nitrate to be detectable?
Buffering agents and salts to control pH are typically used at a few tenths of a percent. If you rubbed lotion on your arm that contained 0.1% of a nitrate, the amount of nitrate deposited would be above the detection threshold of devices like the EN5000 Tabletop Detector, made by Scintex Trace Corp, which can detect nitrates down to the nanogram and picogram level.

THE BOTTOM LINE
The notion that your skin lotion is explosive is ridiculous. But it seems plausible (but not very likely) that your lotions could trigger a false positive on airport detectors.

Do silicones stop other ingredients from working?

Ella inquires: Just wondering – if all sorts of 'cones + glycerine are up in the ingredients list and then followed by other ingredients like vitamins, peptides, natural oils etc., won't they prevent the later from penetrating the skin, thus not making any positive effect by staying on the surface? I have this perception (maybe the wrong one) that silicones sort of coat skin surface, not letting anything in or out. Then if they are on top of the list, other ingredients should be useless... I looked through your wonderful site but only seem to find info about silicones in the context of hair products. But hair is dead and skin is a live organ, so the effect of cones on it might be different? Please correct me if I am wrong. why I am asking... I color my hair at home using brown or dark brown shades. They stain skin around my hair line. I experimented with applying all sorts of moisturizing creams near the hair line beforehand and SURPRISE – those with 'cones (like Olay) work the best in keeping stains away. Sooooo, if you stuff a cream with all sorts of goodies for the skin and then go generous on 'cones for better feeling and gliding application, won't they prevent all the goodies from absorbing, just like they prevent hair color sinking in the skin?... hmmm

The practice of applying a barrier cream before certain chemical processes is well known. For example, petrolatum is used to protect the hair line during application of hair relaxer. We haven't seen a definitive technical answer for why silicone (or other occlusive agents) don't prevent "goodies" from being absorbed, but here's what could be happening.

Silicone takes time to form a film

When delivered from a cream, ingredients like silicones and petrolatum have to be spread across the skin and allowed to dry before they form a barrier film. When you apply a cream containing "goodies" along with silicones, the cream hits the face all at once. The ingredients that will penetrate have time to sink into the skin before all the water evaporates and the silicones set up an occlusive film. When you apply a silicone cream FIRST and then sometime later apply another product (like a hair color) the silicones have had time to set up as a film, and so they do a better job of keeping stuff OUT of the skin. Hence, no staining.

THE BOTTOM LINE

Chemists balance the ingredients in their formulas to make sure that they are delivered properly. If silicones prevented other active agents from doing their job, they would have been phased out by now in favor of something that did a better job.

Is my conditioner giving me acne?

Allison asks...I heard that when you are washing a way conditioner in the shower it comes in contact with your body's skin and may cause clogged pores (same goes if it runs down your face) and cause breakouts. So now I make sure to shower after I wash out the conditioner. Is it ridiculous?

Hmmm, if that's true, some enterprising company should be marketing an acne-free hair conditioner!

3 reasons conditioner won't cause acne

First, your conditioner would have to contain ingredients that have a high comedogencity potential. (Remember that comedogenicity is the measure of how likely a given ingredient, or blend of ingredients, is to cause clogged pores.) Second, the ingredients would have to stick to your skin and not be diluted down as they're rinsed from your hair. (The contact time with your skin would be very brief, so we find that hard to imagine.)

Third, since your entire body is wet from the shower, your skin will have absorbed about as much moisture as it can. Therefore there isn't much drive (aka an osmotic gradient) for the ingredients to be absorbed into your skin as they run down your body toward the drain. We're not saying it's impossible, but it seems very unlikely.

THE BOTTOM LINE

To be safe, you can continue to shower after conditioning, but there seems little reason to fear that your conditioner is causing acne.

Can I get a stronger SPF by doubling my sunscreens?

Erica asks...Does mixing moisturizer SPF 20 and tinted moisturizer SPF 20 make SPF 40?

It's math time!

Common sense chemistry

The easiest way of thinking about it is if you took two of the same sized cups of water and put two drops of blue food coloring dye in each cup. The depth of blue color you'd get in each cup would be the same. What color blue would it be if you then mixed your two cups together? The same color blue. In the analogy, the food coloring is like the active ingredients in your sunscreen/moisturizer, and the water is the inactive ingredients.

One more thing: there MAY be some benefit to using SPF in both products because if you under-apply the first product the second product will help ensure you get enough coverage. In other words, using two SPF twenty products won't give you SPF 40, but it will help ensure you that you apply enough to get to 20. It doesn't matter what the SPF number on the bottle is if you don't apply enough to your skin!

THE BOTTOM LINE

More sunscreen is always better when it comes to protecting your skin. But don't think that you're getting increased SPF protection just because you're using two different products.

What happens when you mix different sunscreens?

Jean asks... I read that wearing two different sunscreens with SPF 20 does not add up to SPF 40, but it will help ensure I to get to 20. I have been wondering, what is the protection factor if the SPFs are not the same? If I wear a moisturizer SPF 30 and then a foundation SPF 15 what does it make?

Here are the guesses that Eugenie put forth in her original question:

• SPF 15, because it's the last applied?

• SPF 30, because it's the first applied or because it's the higher SPF?

• Between SPF 15 and 30, because it's a mix?

• SPF 45, because it's like an addition? (She didn't really think it works like this, but it's an option)

• Greater than SPF 30, because it increases the SPF?

What do you think the answer is?

More sunscreen math

Think of it this way: If you took 1 ounce of SPF 15 lotion and mixed it with 1 ounce SPF 30 lotion, you'd be creating 2 ounces of SPF 22.5 lotion (assuming that there was no interaction between the ingredients, which is not necessarily a good assumption). So, if you applied them at the same time, you could end up with less than 30.

If you applied the SPF 30 first, let it soak into your skin, and then later applied the SPF 15, you may be helping maintain the 30, but that's the best you can hope for.

THE BOTTOM LINE

Sunscreen application doesn't add up linearly. The best thing you can do is to use a high SPF and apply it frequently if you're out in the sun.

Can skin lotions interfere with sunscreens?

Pat asks...Does using facial oils, from certain brands or in general, under a sunscreen affect how good it works? My skin loves certain oils and in spring/summer I use them during the day underneath my sunscreen. I was wondering if it affected the SPF and how well it protects; does the oil dissolve some of the protection if it's a chemical one?

The active ingredients in sunscreens are drugs that can interact with other products.

Sunscreen interactions

There is cause for concern because it is well documented that certain ingredients can interact with sunscreens. Sometimes this interaction is good; sometimes it's not so good. For example, a chemical known as Mexoryl SX can improve SPF by reducing the photo degradation of certain UV absorbers like Parsol 1789. Iron chelators like vitamin C and E can also slow the breakdown of sunscreens. On the other hand, care must be taken when mixing sunscreens with insect repellants; because of interaction with DEET (the stuff that repels the bugs), skin penetration is increased.

THE BOTTOM LINE

It's best not to mix sunscreens and other products. The best approach is to wait 10 or 15 minutes between application of products. If you apply an oil to the skin at the same time as the sunscreen, you are essentially diluting the sunscreen and it won't be as effective. Of course, no matter what technique you use, the key message here is to wear sunscreen!

Why don't they make SPF 200 sunblock?

Ronnie says...I looked for SPF 200 on the internet (the INTERNET for crying out loud!) and I couldn't find a single seller. WTF?

For better or worse the world of sunscreens is still evolving.

Fun with the FDA

The FDA has recently will introduced new limits, making the maximum allowable claimed SPF 50+. Although before this change was flagged there was certainly a race for ever increasing SPF numbers in the USA, we can imagine some brand manager demanding an SPF 200 product in a new product meeting, so why not...? Here are three reasons:

• Cost. Sunscreen agents are expensive

• Aesthetics. Organic sunscreens feel horrible and oily; inorganic suncreens would leave the skin too white

• Diminishing returns. A SPF 15 will block about 94% of UV light, SPF 30 97%, SPF 50 98%, SPF 100 99%.

THE BOTTOM LINE

Rather than looking for SPF 200, you're better off spending your money on a good SPF 50 product and making sure you apply it really well.

Can I become immune to eyeshadow primer?

Erin asks...I have recently noticed that my eye shadows are creasing like crazy, like 3.5 years ago before I started using primers. I used MAC Paintpot for those 3.5 years and the last pot is probably 1.5 years old, but hasn't dried up yet and still has a very creamy consistency. I switched to the sample of Urban Decay Primer potion and that creased as well. I tried not moisturizing my eye area and not putting sunscreen to see if it makes a difference, but it was exact same creasing result. I Googled the phenomenon and found a post from a girl experiencing the exact same thing – she gets immune to the primer after awhile: http://thebeautybrains.com/dbmoT. Any explanation and advice? The UDPP is also 1.5-2 years old at most... don't think it could be the age of the product, as the first paintpot I had lasted me over 2 years and never creased.

We read the post from the other girl experiencing this problem. She's using a Claudia Stevens product and said that "I have used that primer everyday for the last 5 or 6 months, and about 2 weeks ago, I noticed that it started to crease on me."

What's in eyeshadow primer?
Rather than thinking that you're becoming "immune" to the product, our assumption is that something in the product is changing over time. Is there something that these products all have in common that could cause them to stop working over time? Looking at the ingredients (see below), you'll notice that the two most predominant ingredients are isododecane and cyclopentasiloxane, both of which are designed to make the primer more spreadable. But these ingredients have a low vapor pressure, which means they evaporate quickly. That's good, because it means they won't leave a heavy residue on your skin. But it also means that over time there will be less and less of these ingredients left in the product. It's conceivable that as these two ingredients evaporate, the other ingredients don't spread across your skin as well. That could be what's accounting for the "creasing" effect you're seeing.

(To make matters worse, some of these products are sold in tiny flat jars with widemouth openings. This creates a large amount of surface area that can speed up evaporation if the product is open too long or used very frequently.)

It's easy enough to test this theory by buying a new sample of a product that's no longer working for you and using them side by side. If the new product works and the older one doesn't, then it's likely that evaporation is the problem.

Urban Decay ingredients:

Isododecane, Cyclopentasiloxane, Disteardimonium Hectorite, Trimethylsiloxysilicate, Polyethylene, Trihydroxystearin, Triethylhexanoin, Isopropyl Lanolate, Sorbitan Sesquioleate, VP/Eicosene Copolymer, Dimethicone, PEG-40 Stearate, Propylene Carbonate, Phenoxyethanol, Synthetic Beeswax, Propylparaben, Methylparaben, Butylparaben, Ethylparaben, Isobutylparaben

MAC paint pot ingredients:

Isododecane, Dimethicone, Polyethylene, Hydrogenated polyisobutene, Quaternium-90 bentonite, Dimethicone silylate, Octyldodecanol, Silica, Trihydroxystearin, Retinyl Palmitate, Tocopheryl Acetate, Lecithin, Carnauba Wax, Propylene carbonate, Titanium Dioxide, Iron Oxides, Bismuth Oxychloride, Blue 1 Lake, Carmine, Chromium Hydroxide Green, Manganese Violet, Ultramarines, Yellow 5 Al Lake, Triethoxycaprylylsilane, Mica, Chromium oxide greens, Ferric ferroxyanide

Claudia Stevens Makeup Before The Makeup ingredients:

Water, Cyclopentasiloxane, Isododecane, Glyceryl laurate, Beeswax, Polyglyceryl-4 oleate, Stearyl dimethicone, Ethylhexyl stearate, Microcrystalline wax, Talc, Cetyl PEG/PPG-10/1dimethicone, Phenoxyethanol, Ethylparaben, Propylparaben, Methylparaben, Butylparaben, Isobutylparaben, Mica,

Disteardimonium hectorite, Silica, Tocopheryl acetate, Propyl-ene carbonate, Titanium dioxide, Iron oxides.

THE BOTTOM LINE

If this proves to be the case, what can you do about it? Well, you could look for brands that don't have cyclopentasiloxane as the first or second ingredient. Notice that the Mac product has dimethicone, which does not evaporate. Of course that solution is not without potential trade-offs: you may find that the site dimethicone-based products don't spread across your eyelids as easily and then you'll have to make the decision about which is better: a product that keeps working longer but doesn't spread as well or a product that tends to dry up more quickly but gives you a better feel while it does work. The only way to tell for sure is to try a few different products and find the right one for you.

How can I stop my husband from washing with my shampoo?

Connie's question...My husband uses my shampoo as body wash, and it drives me crazy. Can you give me some technical reason to make him stop??

We've always considered shampoo and body wash to be pretty similar. But a 2012 article in the respected publication Cosmetics & Toiletries (http://thebeautybrains.com/uliqp) takes a slightly different position. Does that mean we should agree with Carol or her husband? Read on...

Shampoo versus body wash

The authors of the article (the esteemed Tony O'Lenick and his collaborator Dr. Zhang) point out that "hair cannot be cleansed well with body wash" because "Shampoos were created because hair became rough and damaged when cleansed with soap." While we agree that soap leaves hair feeling less conditioned, we don't think it's accurate to say that hair "can't" be cleaned well with body wash. Perhaps it's more accurate to say that the average body wash will not provide as much conditioning to hair as a good moisturizing (aka 2 in 1) shampoo. But for those who like their hair squeaky clean, body wash will do a fine job.

The authors also posit that "Body wash contains milder surfactant bases than shampoos." While this would have been generally true a few years ago, the increasing popularity of sulfate free shampoos have tended to equalize the mildness of both product types.

On the flip side, the authors point out that using shampoo in place of body wash can on the body can leave the skin with a "slimy feel." Again, if you're used to using deep cleansing body washes, this may be the case. But if you're a fan of Olay type body washes that contain significant levels of petrolatum and other moisturizing agents, then you might enjoy the feel of shampoo.

THE BOTTOM LINE

We're sorry, Connie, but we can't honestly give you any technical evidence to use against your husband. While everyone likes their skin to feel a certain way after cleansing, there's no problem with using shampoo as an occasional substitute for body wash. You might even find that you like it better!

Should I pat my face with water before applying oil?

Judy inquires: In another beauty-related forum, I read the following claim about applying a face oil: "Make sure your face and your hands are slightly damp when applying the oil. Rub the oil between your hands to emulsify slightly, then pat it on your face and massage it in. The oil will help trap the water in. " Is this true? Can the skin really absorb water this way? And if so, is it beneficial in any way?

The quick answer is: it won't hurt, but it won't really help much either.

How moisturizers work

The main moisturizing function of oil is to create a barrier that prevents the moisture in the deep layers of your skin from evaporating. The oil can only lock in the water that's already absorbed by your skin. So, if you've just saturated your skin by taking a shower, then you'll lock in quite a bit of moisture with oil. But if your face is dry and then you just splash it with a little water before applying oil, you're really not helping that much.

Creams and lotions are designed to deliver oil WITH water so you lock in the deeper moisture that's already in your skin AND get a quick hit of surface moisture from the water in the lotion.

What is "emulsify?"

Also, just to clarify, you can't really "emulsify" oil and water just by rubbing them together in your hands. There are many technical definitions of emulsify, but to put it in layperson terms, it means to disperse tiny droplets of one liquid in another liquid. Since oil and water water don't naturally mix, you need a chemical known as an emulsifier (also called a surfactant) allows the two to co-mingle without separating.

THE BOTTOM LINE

There's no need to go through an extra step of patting your face with water. Just make sure you moisturize after cleansing and you'll be fine.

Is it safe to use facial cleanser in the shower?

Kim really wants to know...I used to live next to a cosmetologist and she said that when using face cleanser you are supposed to not do it in the shower because it doesn't have time to work. She also said you should do it in an upwards motion to prevent wrinkles (even though I was a preteen, that's what she taught me at a Mary Kay party). I really like using facial cleanser in the shower. Is it true that it's less effective?

"Regular" facial cleaners (simple surfactant-based face washes) are designed to remove makeup, oil, and dirt. These products don't require any extra time to work, so there's nothing wrong with using them in the shower. However, there are a few specialty products that have special usage requirements.

Neutrogena Oil-Free Acne Wash Facial Cleanser

Should be used twice a day for optimum anti-acne efficacy. So unless you want to shower two times a day, you'll have to use it out of the shower.

Freeze 24-7 Ice Shield Face Facial Cleanser with Sunscreen

This product contains a sunscreen that deposits on your skin as you wash your face; it needs to be left on 1 to 2 minutes before rinsing, which maybe be difficult to do in the shower.

Upwards motion to prevent wrinkles?

Applying a facial wash with an "upwards" motion will not help prevent the causes of aging like photo-aging or the collapse of collagen/elastin fibers. Does your application technique ever make a difference? Yes, in some cases it does. Sunscreens, for example, need to be applied with very even, smooth strokes because they won't work very well if they don't evenly coat the skin. Same thing is true for sunless tanners; if you don't apply them consistently, you'll end up with streaks. Some types of make up have similar application issues.

You need to be careful when applying wrinkle concealing foundations to make sure they fill in those fine lines evenly.

THE BOTTOM LINE
You don't need to apply facial cleanser with upward strokes; however, many facial products do need to be applied uniformly in order to work properly.

Do natural oils smother your skin?

Crystal must know...Here's my big dilemma and it applies to skin, hair, makeup. I love natural oils. My makeup has sunflower oil, castor oil, and beeswax. I put coconut oil on after my nighttime moisturizer. I apply castor oil to my scalp before washing my hair and do deep oil treatments on my hair at times. Now I've read that oils and beeswax are occlusive and don't allow your skin to breathe, and that over the long-term, it will actually damage your skin and allow toxins to go to your liver, because they can't escape through your face. If I'm really not allowing pores to breathe, than castor oil will eventually make my hair fall out, no?

Don't worry, Crystal, using natural oils won't cause your liver to fail.

Occlusive is good for your skin

Most oils (natural oils, mineral oils, and silicones) ARE occlusive – that just means that they can reduce the amount of water that evaporates through your skin. But they don't SEAL the skin in such a way that sweat glands stop working. Your skin doesn't need to breathe; it just needs to be able to perspire so it can regulate your body temperature. Occlusive ingredients in topical cosmetics do not impact how much you perspire, so you don't need to worry. Also, the liver handles getting rid of the toxins. That's not the skin's job.

You do need to worry about ingredients that can contribute to clogged pores, however, because they can lead to acne. There are several sites that allow you to check the comedogenicity rating of ingredients in your products. (Or, just look for products that are labeled non-comedogenic.)

THE BOTTOM LINE

The idea that cosmetics lock in toxins is a common beauty myth. By understanding the science of how your body works it's easy to see that simply can't be true.

Is it okay to hack my lip gloss?

Veronica must know...I have a lipgloss I love, but it is very bright, so I don't wear it every day. This means it has lasted me a long, long time. So long, in fact, that the company has stopped making that variety (Dior's Diorific Plastic Shine, in case you were wondering). The gloss is starting to thicken now, and while it can still be used, it would be easier if it were a bit thinner. Is it possible to thin out a thickened lip gloss?

It's very frustrating when a company discontinues one of your favorite products. But sometimes you just have to let go...

Diluting cosmetics is dangerous
Diluting cosmetics (especially ones used on the lips) is always tricky because you're also diluting the preservative system. Under-preserved cosmetics are dangerous because they can harbor bacteria and fungi that can make you sick. If the product is oil-based instead of water-based, the risk is somewhat lower, but even products that contain no water whatsoever can be contaminated if they come in contact with moist fingers, the environment, etc. (We couldn't find an ingredient list for this product, so it's difficult to tell for sure.) Therefore, we recommend finding a replacement product.

Having said all that, Ally in the Beauty Brains Forum had a good idea that might just save the day for you. She suggests putting the tube into a cup of hot water and leaving it there for awhile. While this might not permanently thin out the product, it certainly could make it flowable enough to apply.

THE BOTTOM LINE
Don't take the chance of challenging a product's preservative system by diluting it. But gently warming it could make it easier to apply.

Do hair removal creams damage skin?

Angela asks...I currently use a hair removal cream (Veet) and have heard people say that over time it can damage your skin. Is this true?

Veet and other hair removal creams work by using thioglycolate to break down the disulfide bonds that hold hair together. (Veet should not to be confused with the mosquito repellant DEET which should never be applied under your arms and in the bikini region. Unless of course your clandestine romantic activities make you prone to mosquito bites in those areas.) Anyway, the chemistry of these hair removal products is similar to how perms and relaxers work.

How do hair removal products affect skin?
Skin has a different amino acid profile than hair. Whereas hair is held together with disulfide bonds that come from relatively high levels of cystine, skin does not have much cystine. Therefore, thioglycolate will not "dissolve" skin the same way it does hair. Now, because of the high pH required to swell the cuticle and let the thioglycolicate do its job, these creams can be irritating to skin. In fact, in its pure form, thioglycolate is very hazardous and should not come into contact with skin at all unless you want to experience burning, reddening, eczema-like dermatitis and bleeding under the skin. (All according to the Material Safety Data Sheet.) But, properly formulated at the right pH and at a low concentration, this ingredient has been sold in hair removal products for many, many years with a good track record. If you follow the company's instructions for testing the product before you use it and if you haven't experienced any burning or irritation, then you're probably fine.

THE BOTTOM LINE
When it comes to reactive personal care products, you should ALWAYS follow the instructions carefully to reduce the chances of any side effects.

Interesting bonus fact: Veet used to be called Neet.

Does Vaseline darken lips?

Sarah says...Does Vaseline darken lips? I've always used it on my lips before I go to bed, but my roommate tells me that it darkens lips because it can be used to get a greater tan – as it is like an oil. Many people are adding their own anecdotal evidence about how it has darkened their lips – but I don't know what to think! As it is, I have moderately dark lips. Is there any scientific proof?

Vaseline is essentially petrolatum (which is closely related to mineral oil) so it's reasonable to assume that they might work the same way. But we were surprised to find very little research on the effect of tanning oils on skin. (We did find studies on tanning accelerators like L-tyrosine, but that's a story for another day...) Still, after much searching, we did find one reputable source that should definitively answer your question.

Why does oil make you tan better?
Everyone seems to know that rubbing baby oil (aka mineral oil) on your skin will make you tan faster and deeper. Many articles claim that mineral oil "attracts" UV rays. But WHY is that? What's really happening? According to a paper we found in the Journal of the American Academy of Dermatology, mineral oil (and similar lubricants) is used in the photo-therapy treatment of psoriasis to enhance the effects of UVB treatment. Apparently the mineral oil smooths scaly skin and decreases the amount of UV radiation that is reflected. Less reflection means skin absorbs MORE UVB rays. And since UVB rays are responsible for tanning, the skin gets darker. That must be how tanning oils work!

Remember, though, that your lips don't tan. So if you're asking about the actual lips themselves, this won't work. But, if you're asking about the skin of your upper lip, yes, it is very possible that putting Vaseline petroleum jelly on it will make it get darker (after exposure to sun).

THE BOTTOM LINE

Vaseline won't make your lips darker from tanning because lips don't produce melanin (the source of sun tan). But Vaseline will moisturize lips, which could give them a darker color.

Smart phones can't detect skin cancer

We've told you before that you shouldn't trust over the counter mole removal products. But what about smart phone apps that help check moles for skin cancer? Are those safe and effective? New data suggest that your phone isn't smart enough to be trusted with this medical diagnosis.

Mole minder apps

In case you haven't seen them, these apps work by taking a photograph of your mole and then applying mathematical formulae to assess their symmetry and color. If the mole matches a certain set of criteria, the app flags it as being potentially pre-cancerous. But dermatologists at the University of Pittsburg Medical Center (http://thebeautybrains.com/fY4yd) tested some of these smartphone apps and found that they missed dangerous moles about one-third of the time!

Relying on your smartphone instead of your dermatologist may not be so smart after all. But the researchers do recommend apps that help you track changes in moles and then remind you to have your doctor look at them. For example, the University of Michigan's UMSkinCheck sends self-exam reminders. The important thing is to have those moles checked!

Do skin lotions work better if you pat instead of rub?

Carol asks...I've always wondered if there is legitimacy to Clarins' claim that by patting their product into your skin, it works better and you skin absorbs it better than rubbing it in. Is this really true? If so, what about all other skincare products out there? Should we be patting instead of rubbing?

We're not familiar with this particular Clarins product, but the notion that lotion will be absorbed better if you pat it on instead of rubbing it on makes no sense. While patting your face may increase blood flow, blood circulation doesn't play a role in the absorption process, because ingredients penetrate the upper layers of skin by diffusing through the channels between skin cells and not by absorption through blood vessels.

A dermatologist discusses skin penetration

Rather than relying on our knowledge of chemistry to answer this one, we decided to consult one of our dermatologist friends. Here's what she had to say in response to the question:

> Hmm, I had to ponder just what might have led Clarins to this idea, and I'm stumped. You see, the outer dead cell layer of the skin (called the stratum corneum) is THE single, main protective barrier for our skin. Once something gets through the stratum corneum, it has a free ride into the rest of the skin, but getting through the stratum corneum is no easy feat – and the act of rubbing or patting is inconsequential.

> To put it in perspective, if it wasn't for the strength of this huge (like biggest organ in the body sort of huge) barrier, all our important body stuff would be leaching out from our skin all day long, and every substance we came into contact would enter. The integrity of this barrier is a big deal for our health, and it takes more than patting or rubbing to impact it. To breach the stratum corneum, you need to assault it with tactics like a facial acid peel that dissolves it entirely, laser vapori-

zation where it goes up in smoke, repetitive stripping with tape until you've pulled it all off (anyone who has had hair removal waxing knows what I mean), or severe irritation that disrupts the components of the stratum corneum, rendering it defective (think dish pan hands).

When we apply skin care products, by either rubbing or patting, our skin care products sloooowly penetrate our stratum corneum by gradually seeping in (a process called diffusion). Again, whether we pat or rub, they aren't going to get through any faster than the stratum corneum will let them.

THE BOTTOM LINE
Patting on lotion instead of rubbing will not make the product penetrate your skin any differently. If Clarins has any data to the contrary, we'd be glad to review it in a future post.

Why does perfume make me sneeze?

Jenny says....I have a few questions about perfumes and fragrances that I think you Brains would do a good job of answering. I get so sneezy when a perfume is sprayed, and then I usually get a headache. However, I don't have this problem with roll-ons as long as I use a light hand. I just discovered Lush's Lust perfume, which I love for its jasmine scent, but bought in the form of a waxy roll-on because of the sneeze factor. However, it doesn't last very long, and I would love to have that sexy, soft smell on me all day, instead of for just an hour or two!

Here are the fragrance-related questions Jenny sent us, along with our answers.

Question 1
How long do "real" perfumes last once you open them? How long do they last if you DON'T open them for years? (My grandma has a ton of super expensive perfumes from the 1990s never opened and wants to regift them! I think they're prime time for the trash can!)

Answer: As a rule of thumb, fragrances will last up to about two years before their scent changes significantly. Fragrances contain reactive chemicals that won't stay stable for dozens of years. Most perfumes are sealed in glass spray bottles, so they're not "opened" in the sense that a jar of cream is opened, because the product is not typically exposed to the air or contamination from your fingers. But, exposure to light and high temperature can shorten the time they will last. So if by "open", you mean removing the perfume bottle from the outer packaging that's protecting it from light, then yes, it will make a difference.

Question 2
Can you buy a few essential oils (like jasmine or gardenia) and dab them on yourself? Or do they need a carrier agent to stick on you and last? How long do essential oils last once opened?

Answer: You certainly can buy pure essential oils and use them on your skin (just make sure you don't choose one that you're allergic to). But fragrances are much more complex than a few simple notes. They are designed in three parts: top notes, which evaporate quickly and give you an initial burst of fragrance; middle notes, which last up to an hour or so; and then the base notes, which sort of anchor the fragrance to your skin and hopefully last all day. Depending on which essential oils you choose, you may only be getting one of these three types of notes. While you might like the smell of essential oils, you certainly won't get the well-rounded long-lasting performance that you will from a properly compounded perfume.

Question 3

Can you dab on a perfume that's meant to be sprayed by unscrewing the cap, or do perfume dabs need to be in an oily carrier to stick?

Answer: Dabbing is a great solution for your sneezing problem. That's because the sneeze attacks are likely caused by the aerosolized alcohol that you're inhaling. That triggers vasodilation in the nose, which in turn makes you sneeze. (The technical term is "vasomotor rhinitis.") If you apply the perfume directly to your skin, the alcohol will still evaporate, but it won't be aerosolized into tiny particles that are more likely to constrict the blood vessels in your nose. If the perfume is sealed in a spray bottle, you might be able to "smother" the spray into a cotton ball before dabbing it on your skin.

Question 4

Can you add perfume to plain lotion? Rubbing something on seems to not trigger the sneezing attacks like spraying something does – I think I'm just a klutz when it comes to doing anything beauty-related – someday I'll figure out how to use a hair straightening iron without burning myself, but that's a lesson for another day!

Answer: We advise against trying to add perfume oil to a lotion. Fragrances have to be carefully selected for the products they're put into to ensure they are compatible. The fragrance you add could affect the preservative system or impact the stability of the lotion by changing the viscosity or color.

THE BOTTOM LINE
You don't have to be allergic to sneeze at perfumes. Dabbing a dollop can save you from sneezing.

Can tweezing eyebrows make you sneeze?

Brow Beaten asks...I tweeze my own eyebrows, and I notice that almost every time I tweeze I start to sneeze. My sister says I'm just imagining it and it doesn't happen all the time, but I thought maybe you could find out.

Dear Brow Beaten, your "tweeze and sneeze" problem is a new question that we've never heard. We weren't able to find any documentation in the technical literature to confirm this effect is real, but we can think of two possible mechanisms that could explain what's happening to you.

Tweeze and sneeze
First, the act of pulling hairs out of your brows could be agitating the follicle and triggering a histamine response. Histamines are chemicals in your body that are released in response to certain injuries. They increase blood vessel permeability, which in turn allows fluid to escape. This reaction leads to a runny nose and watery eyes, and potentially a sneeze.

Another possibility is that the tweezing is causing your eyes to tear up. When this happens, some of the tears may not be making it all they way out of the tear ducts, and they may be draining back down the lacrimal canal inside your nose. This drainage could be "tickling" the cells inside the nasal cavity and causing a sneeze.

THE BOTTOM LINE
Either way, you don't sound crazy to us. Tell your sister there may be a plausible scientific reason for what your experiencing.

Skin toner is important, right?

EA asks…I was wondering what The Beauty Brains thought about the idea that you need to use toner after cleansing in order to restore the skin to its proper pH. I've come around to thinking that this is an outdated beauty idea, but I would love to hear your take on it.

We think "outdated" is a good way to describe it!

What is skin toner and does it restore pH?
Traditional toners consist of witch hazel extract in alcohol (ethanol) which can be drying and irritating to skin. Does this mixture restore skin pH? Well, your skin pH is a result of the skin's acid mantle, a mixture of sebum (skin oils) and sweat that form on the surface of your skin. This acid mantle keeps the pH of your skin at about 4 to 4.5. A slightly acidic pH protects your skin from becoming infected by harmful bacteria. When you wash your skin, you strip away this acid mantle, because cleansers are very good at dissolving oils. However, this is not really a problem, since your skin will regenerate the acid mantle in just a few hours. Toners don't impact the regeneration of the acid mantle and are therefore unnecessary. They may feel refreshing, but you don't need them for the sake of pH balance.

THE BOTTOM LINE
You don't need to buy yet another product just to restore your skin's pH. It will do that on its own very nicely.

Can insect repellant dissolve tights?

Nancy says...A friend of mine put on OFF (repellant) all over her legs; she was using the aerosol form. And then she put in black tights. A while later we noticed that her tights/stockings were super blotchy. It was completely ruined. What happened?

Boy, this sure sounds like an urban legend, doesn't it?

The danger of dissolvable DEET
The active ingredient in OFF is DEET, which is an effective solvent that can dissolve rayon, spandex, and other synthetic fabrics. Her tights are probably made from some combination of natural and synthetic fibers like nylon or acetate. She should switch to all cotton tights or a non-DEET containing product. Or else just stay indoors.

THE BOTTOM LINE
Surprisingly, insect repellant can dissolve tights. Who would have thought?

Do breast implants grow mold?

Michelle asks...Is it true mold grows in breast implants after 10 years in both saline and silicone?

We consulted with one of the industry's experts on this subject: cosmetic plastic surgeon, and friend of the Beauty Brains, Dr. Anthony Youn.

Celebrity Cosmetic Surgeon

You might know Dr. Youn through his blog Celebrity Cosmetic Surgery; it's the definitive site to learn about who's had a little nip and tuck in Hollywood. He's also the author of a highly entertaining and informative book called "In Stiches" about the behind the scenes world of plastic surgery.

Moldy breast implants?

We forwarded Michelle's question to Dr. Youn and here's what he had to say:

> It's not true. Mold does not grow on breast implants unless they were inserted in a nonsterile manner or the saline used to fill an implant was contaminated. Typically, saline implants are filled directly from a sterile IV bag, and so the chances of contamination are nearly zero. It's considered a closed system. When saline is inserted into the implants in an open system, such as when saline used to fill an implant is placed in an open bowl, then the risks of contamination, in particular mold growth inside the implant, is higher.

THE BOTTOM LINE

The "shelf life" of breast implants is not impacted by mold and fungus. Looks like another beauty myth busted!

Hair care questions

Do salon products use better quality ingredients?

Chris asks...Talking with my hairdresser, she suggested that I use Oribe products, which they sold at the salon. I told her that I was very pleased with switching off between my Aveeno and Garnier products, and asked her what was so special about this Oribe line of hair care that justified the price, outside of smell and a pretty bottle. To this she told me that Oribe products are made with premium grades of basic ingredients such as sulfates and silicone. And that the 'cones in drugstore products were made with cheaper, inferior, weaker silicone and sulfates. However, I always thought that good old dimethicone would be the same bought in bulk by any company, for any product. Or are there truly different grades of quality?

This question comes from a discussion in our Forum where Chris commented that her stylist "looked like I punched her in the face when I told her I use drug store brands." Thanks for making us smile, Chris.

Higher cost does not mean higher quality

As you suspected, your stylist is a bit misinformed. As we've explained before, stylists are often at the mercy of whatever they're told by the salon companies, which is often inaccurate, to say the least. In this particular case, it is NOT true that salon products buy higher quality grades of cosmetic ingredients than companies that make retail products. Having spent over 40 years in the beauty industry, we've worked with all the major suppliers of cosmetic raw materials and we can assure you that there is not a two-tiered pricing structure for retail and salon.

But there are differences between ingredients

It is true, however, that you can purchase better types of ingredients. For example, we wrote how the more expensive Sodium Cocoyl Isethionate (SCI) is milder than the less expensive Sodium Lauryl

Sulfate (SLS). And it's true that you can buy different grades of a given raw material that may function differently. For example, a high molecular weight dimethicone can condition better than a lower weight of the same material. BUT, and this is the important part, all these different ingredients (and different versions of ingredients) are available to anyone in the industry who wants to purchase them.

Some ingredients are exclusive

So are we saying that there are no ingredients that are exclusive to certain companies? No, we're not saying that at all. There are (at least) two situations where a company may be able to purchase (or at least use) a type of ingredient that is not available to any other company. The first situation occurs when a company has an exclusive purchasing agreement with a supplier.

It's not uncommon in the industry for a raw material supplier to go to a beauty company and say something like, "Hey, I will give you exclusive rights to this raw material if you can guarantee me you will buy a kabillion pounds every month for the next 20 years." However, and again this is the important point, this kind of arrangement only works when the beauty company is able to buy a large enough quantity of the raw material to justify the deal.

In other words, big companies who will buy a lot of a raw material are given the opportunity for these exclusive arrangements. And guess what? Most salon brands are not big enough to justify these kind of deals. If a large manufacturer who owns salon brands (like P&G, Unilever or L'Oreal) enters into an exclusive raw material agreement, they're likely to leverage that raw material across as many brands as possible to make the use of it more profitable. The small salon companies just can't afford to do this.

Patents can be exclusive

The other situation which can lead to one company having an exclusive use of a raw material involves patented technology. If a company has patented a certain application for an ingredient or combination of ingredients, they may have exclusive rights to the use of that ingredient under certain circumstances. But guess who has the deep pockets required to research and develop new patented technologies? That's right, it's not the small exclusive salon brands.

THE BOTTOM LINE

With all due respect to stylists (who really are haircutting artists and not technical gurus) salon companies do not buy better grades of raw materials than companies who make drugstore or other retail brands. So, spending more money on salon products does NOT guarantee you're getting a better quality product.

Does hair grow faster upside down?

Julia's gem... Is it true that hanging your head over the bed for five minutes a day helps hair grow faster because of the blood rushing to your head?

Sorry Julia, but that's a myth. All that will help you grow is a head-ache!

Hang your head and cry

Hair growth isn't just about blood circulation. It has to do with the biochemistry of what goes on in your follicles, the tiny tubes beneath the scalp where the roots of the hair are. There are a couple of drugs that help prevent hair loss (like Minoxidil and Propecia) but for most people the best way to get longer hair is by reducing breakage and splitting.

Can baking soda make shampoo work better?

Bonnie begs to know...I recently read on Eco-Chick and a couple of other places that adding a little baking soda to shampoo can help get rid of styling residue and other gunk in your hair. How does this work? Is it safe for hair?

Adding baking soda to shampoo is a very persistent beauty myth. Using baking soda as a shampoo substitute (i.e., as a dry shampoo) does make some sense because the powder can absorb oil and some surface dirt. But will adding baking soda to shampoo really result in better cleansing? There are three potential reasons why this might work:

3 Ways Baking Soda MIGHT Clean Your Hair

Enhanced detergency

Detergents, which belong to a chemical classification known as surfactants, work because they have both oil and water soluble properties. Baking soda, on the other hand, is a water soluble salt which doesn't really have provide any detergency. You can easily demonstrate this by dissolving some in water and adding a drop of oil. If the baking soda was good at washing away oil, it would disperse the oil droplet. (But it doesn't.)

Increased abrasion

If you had some very insoluble substance stuck in your hair that shampoo would not remove, like chewing gum, the gritty texture of baking soda might help physically abrade it. But for the common types of soil that you will find in your hair (sebum and styling residue), you don't need this increased abrasion.

Raising the pH to dissolve styling residue

At first glance this approach potentially makes the most sense. Styling polymers are neutralized with acid to make them less water-soluble (that's why they can hold your hair in high humidity). One way to get rid of styling gunk is to make it more soluble by raising the pH. Since the pH of a baking soda solution is about 9, this could work, right?

That, as they say, is a testable proposition. So we added a 1/8 teaspoon of baking soda to 1/2 ounce of the shampoo we're currently testing (the new Mark Anthony Oil of Morocco Argan Oil shampoo). Then we measured the pH using test strips.

The test strips showed that the initial pH is pretty close to 7, which is neutral. After adding a good slug of baking soda, the pH strip turned slightly darker; it looks like it went up to about 8 or 8.5. Unfortunately, this much of a pH increase won't provide much cleaning boost to the shampoo, because baking soda is a weak base, and it won't do a very good job of neutralizing the weak acids present in the styling resins.

THE BOTTOM LINE

While adding baking soda to your shampoo won't hurt your hair, it also won't help much. So if you like to do this and you think it gives you a little bit of an edge in cleaning power, go for it. But, if you're going to run out and buy a 50 gallon barrel of baking soda just because you think it's critical for clean hair, then save your money.

Does your own sebum protect your hair?

Annie asks...It's widely known that coconut oil can reduce the swelling of the hair shaft when applied before washing. Does your own sebum provide the same protection against 'hygral fatigue' as coconut oil does?

We've never seen data on sebum in this regard since it's not typically applied to hair as an ingredient. However, we doubt it works as well as coconut oil for these reasons:

Sebum doesn't have the same composition as coconut oil

Sebum is composed of a variety of fatty acids (http://thebeautybrains.com/CLQ8f), including lauric acid, which is the main fatty acid (~50%) in coconut oil. However, lauric acid is "a relatively minor sebaceous fatty acid." That means sebum doesn't contain as much of the "goodies" as coconut oil.

It's hard to get the right dose of sebum

Your scalp produces a relatively small amount of sebum, and it has to "wick" its way along all your hair fibers to be uniformly distributed. That means the ends of the hair (which are most damaged and need the most conditioning) will get the least sebum. Therefore, sebum won't be as effective as a high dose of coconut oil that you can apply uniformly through your hair.

THE BOTTOM LINE

To get enough sebum to treat your hair you'll probably have to harvest massive quantities of it from friends and family as they sleep, and then you'll have to fractionally separate out the lauric acid. It might be easier just to buy a jar of coconut oil. PS, we love the term "hygral fatigue."

Is It okay to use rinse out conditioner as a leave in?

DeAnne asks...Is it okay to use a regular conditioner as a leave in conditioner? I have long, thick wavy hair that needs to be weighed down. Any recommendations or ingredients to look for?

Rinse off and leave-on products are formulated differently for a reason. Almost any oily material will provide conditioning when left on the hair. But a special kind of ingredient is required to ensure that conditioning agents will "stick" to hair during rinsing.

Two kinds of conditioning agents
There are two tricks that chemists use to deposit ingredients on hair. One is called "dilution deposition", which works well for silicones and some oils. In this approach, the ingredients "fall out" of solution when rinse water hits the product. The other approach is called "charge deposition", which requires conditioners known as "quaternary ammonium" compounds or quats for short. Quats have a positive charge, so they are attracted to the negative sites on damaged hair. One issue with quats, though, is that they are typically chloride salts and can be irritating to your skin. Because of this potential irritation issue, some quats that are used in rinse off products should not be used in products that are left in contact with the skin. Cetrimonium chloride is one such example: it can't be used at more than 1% in a leave on product. Because the average consumer has no way of knowing which ingredients will be irritating (and at what concentrations the ingredients are used at) there is some risk in leaving a rinse out conditioner in your hair.

THE BOTTOM LINE
If you choose to experiment with leaving rinse out products in your hair, be mindful that you may experience increased skin irritation.

Are micro-mist steamers really good for hair?

Cher asks...I recently heard of this micro mist steamer hair treatment and how it's supposedly better than regular steamers or heat hair treatments. Can anyone please clarify this issue for me?

This mister does appear to be an effective Extraction Tool. The problem is the only thing that it's extracting is hard earned money from your wallet.

What is a micro mist steamer hair treatment?

An ultrasonic steamer like the Micro Mist from Takara Belmont (http://thebeautybrains.com/hd1TU) generates cool steam, which supposedly swells the hair shaft and allows treatments to penetrate better. In reality, you don't need any expensive device to achieve this same swelling effect – just wetting hair with water causes it to swell. (In fact, too much swelling is not good. Perms, relaxers and coloring processes can swell the hair shaft to the point of damage.)

According to the company, you need to spend big bucks on their machine because it uses "ultrasonic vibrations to emit an enormous quantity of microscopic water particles that permeate deep into hair follicles." These water droplets are supposedly smaller than "conventional" misting or steaming products, so the water penetrates the hair better. Unfortunately, regular water (misted or not) has no trouble penetrating to the cortex of hair, so you don't need to pay for a special treatment to receive this benefit.

Takara Belmont says that using their Mister "creates a sensation for the customer that is often referred to as smooth and relaxing...the Mist emitted is an impressive visual that will get noticed and talked about in your salon environment." There maybe some aesthetic benefits to this treatment, but will not make hair care products work any better.

THE BOTTOM LINE
While it may feel very indulgent and pampering to have this treatment done in a spa, from a technical perspective, this product is not "mist-er right" for your hair.

Does Vaseline lengthen lashes?

Alyssa asks...I've read a lot of articles and watched many Youtube videos claiming that applying Vaseline to your eyelashes and eyebrows every night before sleep helps to lengthen them. I wonder if it's true? I know eyes are sensitive organs, so wouldn't the chemicals in Vaseline, in this case Petroleum Jelly or mineral oil, enter the eyes and cause harmful health effects?

You're not alone in your question about petroleum jelly helping eyelashes and eyebrows grow. We've seen that question a number of times.

Hair growth is hard

Unfortunately, this question goes in the category of beauty myth. There is no plausible technical rationale why petroleum jelly (also known as petrolatum) would have any effect on hair growth whatsoever. So why is this myth so pervasive? Our hunch is that women have applied this to their eyelashes and eyebrows and seen an apparent thickening effect. In other words, just like mascara, this oily substance can make lashes stand out and look thicker. Since the oil also increases reflectance and shine, it may make the lashes appear more dramatic. In theory, it could even be providing a little lubrication to lashes which helps keep them from falling off so soon.

Is petrolatum safe?

So if you do like this effect, is it safe to apply these products close to your eyes? Yes, because the notion that petrolatum and mineral oil cause cancer is just a myth. These ingredients are very safe, because they are highly purified. The molecules are too large to penetrate through the skin and into your bloodstream. Of course, as with any product, you should keep it out of the eye itself. Even the mildest products can have a stinging effect.

THE BOTTOM LINE

Petrolatum is safe for use around the eye, but there is no technical reason why it should help your eyelashes grow longer.

Why does my relaxer stop working?

Shawna says... What can you tell us about relaxer reversion? Sometimes when I have my hair straightened, it goes back to being curly and wavy. What's happening?

To answer Shaniqua's question, we consulted with one of the greatest relaxer experts in the world, Uyi Woghiren, Chief Chemist of Universal Ideas and Concepts, Inc. Here's what Dr. Woghiren had to say on the topic of relaxer reversion:

What cases relaxer reversion?
As Shawna correctly pointed out, reversion refers to the hair returning to a curly or wavy state after being straightened. Even though this is a very common problem, the causes of reversion are not well understood by most people.

As you know, relaxing the hair requires breaking down the chemical bonds, usually with a high pH material such as cream containing sodium, calcium, or lithium hydroxide. These hydroxide creams can be applied by a stylist, a friend, or by yourself. After application of the relaxer into the hair, it is then straightened with a comb. After straightening is completed, the hair is shampooed, conditioned, and styled. Reversion occurs in a few weeks, usually after one or two shampooings, when the hair begins to revert to its original "S" shape. When they experience this problem, most people blame the product. You'll hear women say something like, "Don't use that brand of relaxer, because it causes reversion." In reality, the answer is not that simple. There are actually two key causes of relaxer reversion.

Reason #1: Relaxer is not strong enough
A good relaxer has over 2% hydroxide concentration. Anything less than 2% will not truly straighten hair. Furthermore, some relaxers are formulated with excessive oils or other ingredients that can interfere with the penetration of the hydroxide active. These ingredients reduce the straightening effect.

Reason #2: Relaxer is not left on the hair long enough

This is quite common for home kits, where the product is being applied by someone who is not a trained stylist. However, even trained stylists may remove the product too quickly through mis-judgment or if if the client is starting to show signs of scalp burning.)

Of course, regardless of the cause, it's always easy to blame the product. But the truth is, most incidences of reversion are due to poor application rather than a bad product.

THE BOTTOM LINE

While it's easy to blame the product, in the case of relaxer reversion, it's more likely that "operator error" is the cause of the problem.

Is hairspray for thick hair just a myth?

RaeAnn asks...I love styling my hair, but it seems when I use hairspray (even the kind that is for thick hair), my style always lets me down. So is there way for thick hair to stay just as I styled it, or is it just science fiction?

That's a tough question to answer, because it depends on what kind of style you're trying to achieve.

Styling science

If you're trying to keep your hair straight, hair spray, gels, and mousses can be pretty effective, especially when used with heat styling tools. But if your hair is very thick and heavy and you're looking for a high degree of tight curl retention, then you're likely to be disappointed with gels and mousses. Look for hairsprays that do not contain water. They do a better job holding your hair, because they don't cause curl droop. (Water containing hair sprays cause curl to relax as soon as they make contact with the hair. That's because the hydrogen bonds that hold the curl are reset by water.)

THE BOTTOM LINE

Water-free hairspray is the best product to lock curls in thick, wavy hair.

Can Damage Travel Up My Hair Shaft?

Mary wonders…I was the victim of a bad hair dye accident (apparently they used the wrong activator, not that I would know), resulting in my hair being dry, damaged and breaking off. It is now more than a year later, and I am still trying to grow out the damage; however, I have only partially trimmed the damaged lengths, because I want to keep the length of my hair. I've heard that hair damage can travel up your hair if you don't cut off all the damage. Is this true? Will I actually cause more damage to my hair by trying to retain the length rather than taking the plunge and going short?

To answer your question, we have to explain a little about hair biology.

The science of hair structure
The technical literature shows that when hair absorbs water, it swells, which causes the upper layer of the cuticle to buckle and crack. Any type of damage that increases the amount of water that the hair absorbs can only make this worse. So, if chemical processing has left the ends of your hair more porous, they will absorb more water and therefore the damage is more likely to increase. If you have actual split ends, then it's even worse. As the hair undergoes multiple cycles of wetting and drying, the split can propagate up the shaft. It's the same principle as a crack in a sidewalk that spreads over time as water and ice split it even further.

What's the solution for over-processed hair?
You could stay ahead of the damage by just trimming a little bit each time. You might also be able to offset some of the increased damage by treating hair with a penetrating oil, like coconut oil, that will essentially water-proof your hair from the inside out.

THE BOTTOM LINE
If left untreated, hair damage can become progressively worse. Make sure you always condition hair to protect it from excessive brushing and combing and use a coconut oil treatment on occasion.

How long do eyelashes last?

Missy has a question about hair loss...Why do we lose 100 hairs a day, and is it true that eyelashes have a lifespan of 150 days?

The answer to both questions lies in understanding the cycles of hair growth.

Why do we lose 100 hairs each day?

Hair goes through three different stages as it grows: Anagen, Catagen and Telogen phases. The Anagen phase is the active growth phase. This stage can last a up to 4 to 6 years for scalp hair and can produce scalp hairs that are three feet or longer. The Catagen stage follows the Anagen stage. This is basically a transitional stage, which means the follicle is slowing down production of the hair. Not much happens here. The third stage is the Telogen, or resting, stage. The hair stops growing and just sits there in the follicle. When the cycle starts all over again with Anagen phase, the old hair is pushed out by the new hair.

The follicles all run on different cycles, so at any given time some percentage of your hair is in some stage of each one of these three phases. That's why on any given day you can lose up to about 100 hairs – because about 100 of the follicles are in a late telogen phase, where they are shedding the fiber.

What can you do about hair loss?

Because this hair growth/shedding cycle is hardwired into your biology, there's nothing you can do about it. The best you can do is take care of the hair while it's still on your scalp to prevent it from breaking off prematurely. Remember, unlike skin cells, hair does not regenerate its surface once it has grown out. That means any damage you do to hair builds up over time. Every time you wash your hair, it causes the hair shaft to swell and contract a little bit. This process can cause the cuticles to crack, leaving your hair susceptible to even greater damage. So, while it sounds obvious, the best things you can do for your hair are to limit exposure to washing/drying/combing damage and to use a good conditioner to lubricate the hair.

What about eyelashes?

There are two different types of hairs: Terminal and Vellus. Terminal hairs, like scalp hairs, are thicker and have a longer growing cycle. These are the hairs you have to cut because they get too long. Vellus hairs are short hairs (a millimeter or less), they are very fine, and they have a very short life cycle. Eyelashes are vellus hairs and have a active growing period of only about a month. They then spend several weeks in catagen/telegen phases, so your estimate of 150 days for they life cycle of an eyelash sounds about right.

THE BOTTOM LINE

All hairs, even eyelashes, grown in a biologically pre-determined pattern. You can expect your eyelashes to last about 5 months before they are replaced by new hairs.

How is makeup setting spray different than hair spray?

Debby says...I'd love to see a comparison of makeup "setting" sprays like Urban Decay All Nighter Long-Lasting Makeup Setting Spray and and plain ol' hairspray.

Ask and ye shall receive. There are (at least) three important differences between hairsprays and makeup setting sprays.

Aerosol versus nonaerosol
The best hairsprays are in aerosol form, because they can be water free. (Water causes your curls to droop because it relaxes hydrogen bonds.) Fortunately, water is good for your skin, so non-aerosol make up setting sprays are perfectly fine. That's good, because you certainly wouldn't want to blast your face with an aerosol spray from close range.

Spot welds versus facial film
Hairsprays are designed to do one thing very well: deliver a fine spray of hair holding polymers. These tiny drops of polymers run down your hair until they get to the intersection where two hair shafts meet. At that spot, they dry to form a tiny little weld point that holds the two hair shafts together. Your hair style is held in place by the effect of thousands of these tiny droplets on thousands of hair shafts.

Make up sprays, on the other hand, need to deliver a more uniform film across your entire face. They can't be as "fluid" as hairspray droplets, or it would drip off your face. Therefore, they contain a much higher degree of solids then hairsprays.

Crunch versus non-crunch
The holding polymers used in hairsprays need to form a very rigid spot weld to hold your hairs in place. Makeup setting sprays need to form a less crunchy, light holding film. That means these formulas contain more emollient type materials. On the ingredient list below you'll see materials like Polyhydroxystearic Acid and Isononyl Isononanoate that are not used in hairsprays.

All Nighter long-lasting makeup setting spray ingredients

Aqua (Water), SD-Alcohol 39-C, Polyhydroxystearic Acid, Isononyl Isononanoate, Ethylhexyl Isononanoate, Sodium Co-camidopropyl PG-Dimonium Chloride Phosphate PVP, Phenoxyethanol, Caprylyl Glycol, Methyl Diisopropyl Propionamide, Dimethicone PEG-7 Phosphate, PPG-3 Benzyl Ether Myristate, Gluconolactone, Sodium Benzoate, Glycereth-5 Lactate, Methyl Methacrylate Cross Polymer, Aloe Barbadensis Leaf Juice, Fragrance.

THE BOTTOM LINE

In some cases, companies will sell a similar formula across different product types. But make up setting sprays really do need to be different than hairsprays. We're not saying that you necessarily need to spend $30 on Urban Decay's 4 ounce product, but don't try and save a few dollars by using your typical hairspray to set your makeup.

Can I dilute my Shampoo?

Faith must know...Do you have to wash your hair with SLS or sodium laureth sulfate to get buildup out of your hair? Is there a milder detergent? Also, I dilute my shampoo, because SLS is harsh, with water - 1 cup. I use a medium amount that I would use for my hair. Does that make it less effective, or does it still have ability to cleanse my hair?

SLS and SLES are among the strongest cleansers, but almost any shampoo will do a decent job of cleaning hair. You could try starting with the "weakest" cleansers first, like a baby shampoo or a sulfate free system. If those don't work to your satisfaction, then you'll have to step up to a stronger clarifying product.

Detrimental dilution
Diluting shampoo will definitely make it a less effective cleanser, which may or may not cause problems for you. If you have short hair, or if you're just shampooing to refresh your style without doing any serious cleaning, then adding water to a bit of shampoo could work very well. But in other cases, like the following examples, diluting shampoo is likely to cause problems:

• You have long long hair

• Your hair is really dirty from sweat and oil.

• You're a heavy user of styling products, especially hairspays and gels, because they contain partially neutralized resins that are less water soluble and are therefore harder to remove.

• You're using Dandruff shampoo. By diluting the active ingredient, you won't be getting the full benefit from the drug product.

• You're using conditioning shampoos 2 in 1s and other conditioning shampoos, which use a "dilution deposition" mechanism to deliver conditioning agents to the hair. If you're pre-diluting the shampoo you may be reducing its ability to condition your hair while it cleanses.

• You may also find that your conditioner doesn't work as well if you dilute the shampoo, because some strongly ionic shampoos can help positively charged conditioners deposit better.

THE BOTTOM LINE

There's nothing wrong with experimenting with shampoo dilution. Just be prepared to rewash your hair if you don't get the effect that you want. And of course, never dilute your shampoo by adding water to the bottle, because that can impair the preservative system, which could result in microbial contamination.

Part 4: Green Products - Green Or Just Greenwashed?

Green products are one of the hottest trends in beauty today. But do you know what terms like "natural" and "organic" really mean? Most people don't know so it's easy for unscrupulous companies to take advantage of you by over-charging you for green-washed product. This chapter helps you understand what green really means in the world of beauty science.

General questions

How can you tell if beauty companies are truly "green"?

Belinda asks...What is the definition of a green product according to you?

As you know if you read our article on the Huffington Post (http://thebeautybrains.com/HeSoq), we don't really believe there IS a good definition of a green product. (Or a "natural" or "organic" product for that matter.) The best definition we've seen involves the sustainability guidelines established by the Global Reporting Initiative (GRI).

How can you tell if a cosmetic company is sustainable?
The GRI is a Netherlands-based organization that has established guidelines for companies who wish to report their impact on the environment. The report covers a number of factors that determine a product's environmental impact, including the following:

• Raw Materials (chemicals and packaging)

• Water sources (including amount recycled)

• Biodiversity (how well they protect the ecosystem)

• Greenhouse gas emission (CO_2 and ozone depleting substances)

• Chemical waste (total amount as well as initiatives to mitigate environmental effects)

Even though these are just a few of the areas covered by the G3 report, it's easy to see that this definition of "green" goes far beyond just asking, "Are you using plant-derived ingredients instead of nasty synthetic chemicals?"

THE BOTTOM LINE
If you want to know if the products you're buying are "green", then you should find out if the company that makes them files a GRI G3

report. (Click here to search the GRI database for reports: http://thebeautybrains.com/f1fPO).

5 reasons cosmetic companies continue to greenwash

According to this article on Cosmetics Design, (http://the beautybrains.com/2KLFR) greenwashing is going to get a lot harder in the natural cosmetic segment, and integrity is of utmost importance. We have to respectfully disagree. Here are 5 reasons that companies will continue to greenwash for a long time.

True natural consumers are still a small market segment

While the natural cosmetic market (http://thebeautybrains.com /cs3iH) is a growing one, it still represents only about 10-15% of the total cosmetic industry. So the biggest manufacturers won't significantly change their best selling formulas just to get a piece of this smaller market. They will, however, add an extract here and there to capture a portion of that market. Greenwashing at its best.

All-natural cosmetics do not work as well

It's just a fact: when you restrict the palette of ingredients you can use to create your formulations, you are at a disadvantage against cosmetic formulators who don't have those restrictions. Sure, you can make products that work; they just won't work as well as the standard cosmetic products. And when it comes to what cosmetics consumers buy, there is no question. Consumers buy products that work. They might say they want all natural or green beauty products, but this is secondary to their desire to have products that work.

Consumers don't know the difference

Another factor that keeps greenwashing around is that consumers do not understand (or care) about the difference between greenwashed products and truly all-natural products. Unless a consumer has a degree in chemistry or otherwise has some insider knowledge about cosmetics, they will not know whether a product is greenwashed or not. They may learn what is greenwashed by reading something on the Internet, but this will not be the majority of cosmetics. As long as the label looks like an all-natural product, most consumers will believe it.

Greenwashing keeps costs down

Cosmetic companies are in the business of making money. They may have secondary goals of sustainability or helping the planet, but when it comes down to it, Burt's Bees is just as interested in making money as Proctor and Gamble. And there is no question that a greenwashed cosmetic costs less than an all-naturally formulated cosmetic. As long as profit is a motivation, greenwashed cosmetics will continue to be made.

There are no required standards

Finally, the fact that there are no official government standards for cosmetic products means that any company can pretty much make any product and call it natural. Maybe they can't put a special organic seal or certified label, but that doesn't matter to most of the cosmetic-buying consumers. Until there are governmental standards that everyone in the industry has to follow, there will be greenwashing.

THE BOTTOM LINE

The main reason why greenwashing will continue...It works (at least for now). And until sales of products that claim they are natural and organic without actually being so, companies will continue to make those products.

What do certified organic and cruelty free symbols mean?

Cheri asks...I've been purchasing shampoos that are either organic sulfate paraben free or sulfate paraben free. I purchase these shampoos because sulfate shampoos makes my scalp itch with some slight irritation. I have a question on the symbols I see on the labels of shampoo products and I am interested in knowing what makes a product different than the other. These are symbols or logos such as Certified Organic Ingredients, rabbit ears that state "cruelty free", and the USDA Organic logo.

The logos for USDA Organic and Certified Organic are both controlled by the United States Department of Agriculture's National Organic Program (NOP). (Note: These standards were created for food products, but cosmetics are entitled to use them also.)

100% Organic or just Organic
100% products must contain ONLY organically produced ingredient AND processing aids (not including water and salt). "Organic" products have to contain at least 95% organically produced ingredients. Products that meet this criteria may use the USDA organic logo on their packaging and in advertising.

Less than 70% organic
Products that contain less than 70% organically derived ingredients cannot use USDA organic logo. They may, however, state that they contain "Certified Organic Ingredients" on the product's information panel (on back of the pack).

Cruelty free
The Cruelty Free rabbit ears logo is from PETA (People for the Ethical Treatment of Animals) and is officially known as the "Caring Consumer bunny logo". Products that meet PETA's requirements (meaning that they were produced without testing on animals) can display this logo.

THE BOTTOM LINE

Unfortunately, none of these logos will help you select products that are free of ingredients which will make you itch. If you know you're sensitive to sulfates or parabens, you'll just have to keep an eye on the ingredient list to make sure you're not buying products that contain those chemicals.

We're sick of "Chemical Free" products!

Here at the Beauty Brains, as well as other enlightened places across the beauty blog-o-sphere, there's been a lot of discussion lately about the use of the term "chemical free" as it relates to cosmetics.

There's no such thing as "chemical free"

As our science-savvy readers know, there is no such thing as "chemical free." Everything is a chemical, even water. A chemical free product would be nothing but an empty bottle. Wait a minute; it wouldn't even have a bottle, because bottles are made of chemicals too! Nonetheless, not only do manufacturers insist on using this term, but a frighteningly large number of consumers have embraced it as well.

But rather than just continue to whine about how asinine the term is, we've decided we should do something about it: we should find a better alternative.

What does "chemical free" mean to you?

Of course, before we can identify an alternative phrase, we have to understand what is being implied by the companies spreading the message and what is being inferred for the consumers who have embraced it. We don't know if anyone has already articulated this, but it seems obvious that "chemical free" is a short hand way of expressing that the product is safe to use and good for the environment.

THE BOTTOM LINE

Assuming that safety is at least part of the concern, then what could be a good potential alternative for chemical free? How about something like "certified safe?" (Yeah, we know, then we have to deal with who's responsible for certification. But it's just an example.) So that's our challenge to you, the Beauty Brains community: help us brainstorm another term that could replace "chemical free."

Can natural extracts preserve cosmetics?

Cindy says...Can natural extracts really preserve Shea Moisture's Organic Raw Shea Butter Moisture Retention Shampoo?

We were skeptical that the natural extracts contained in the product would provide sufficient protection against microbial growth. However, we decided to seek out expert advice on the preservation question. So, we consulted a professional microbiologist who has worked on shampoo and conditioner formulas.

Natural extracts can preserve products
According to our consultant (who admittedly knows much more microbiology than any of the Beauty Brains), these extracts MAY be preserving the product.

"Yes, rosemary extract has been known to posses antimicrobial properties, and antioxidants will act as preservative boosters. However, I am not very familiar with the other two extracts. They are one of a number of "natural" or preservative free options that are getting a great deal of attention. The argan oil, although not in a completely anhydrous formulation, may also assist with creating a synergistic effect. Therefore, it is possible that there may not be any additional preservatives."

However, her opinion does come with a caveat:

"...while I have not personally tried any of them; I would expect there to be an evident aesthetic impact if used at sufficient enough levels to be efficacious."

We should also point out that natural extracts may be perfectly adequate for home formulators who are making small batches of product in their kitchens where they have total control over the cleanliness of the equipment. When it comes to large scale manufacturing, it becomes much more difficult to ensure product preservation because of the so-called "house bugs" that can grow in the cracks and crevices of manufacturing tanks, pumps, and transfer lines.

THE BOTTOM LINE

Based on this additional information, we have to admit the possibility that this formula is adequately preserved with the ingredient list that has been provided. We are, after all, skeptical scientists, not knee jerk natural product naysayers. While we're not completely convinced, all it would take is a look at the formula and the results of any microbial challenge testing that was done on the product to know for sure.

See the effort on the top.

How can we reduce animal testing?

Nicky wants to know... What's the latest scoop on animal testing? I'm still worried that cosmetic companies abuse too many bunnies and such.

Nicky, your question could not have come at a better time. We just read a press release from the Scientific Advisory Committee of the European Center for the Validation of Alternative Methods (also known as ECVAM) who announced that there are 5 new methods of testing skin and eye irritation that previously had to be done on rabbits. That means that products like hand soaps, face creams, and make up (among many, many others) can now be safely formulated and tested without harming a single hair on a hare.

But it gets better

One test mimics human skin so well that it will COMPLETELY replace testing on rabbits. Two of the other tests can identify severe eye irritants, which will eliminate the need for live rabbit eye test. And, another new test for skin allergies will cut animal testing in half, saving up to 240,000 mice. All these test methods came about as a result of joint work between the US and the European Union. Thanks guys!!

THE BOTTOM LINE

We're thrilled to see that effective, scientifically valid alternatives to animal testing are becoming increasingly popular in the cosmetic industry. And that means that in the near future Nicky won't have to wonder if any furry little creatures gave their lives to test her favorite eyeshadow, lipgloss or blush.

Do organic preservatives really work?

Cathy asks...I recently read about this organic preservative (Arobo-cide.) I emailed the company (active micro) and they provided me with the information and testing along with their formulation for the testing. Has anyone tried using this in their lotions? I would love to use in my current organic formulation.

It's interesting to watch this debate over safety versus efficacy of ingredients. It seems like some of the greatest debate is in the area of preservatives.

Safety concerns drive development of new preservatives

As we all know, parabens, one of the most common preservatives in cosmetics, are under scrutiny because of concerns over potential carcinogenicity. It's a good thing that the proper research is being done to make sure these ingredients are safe; however, at the time of this writing the best data says that there is no issue with the ingredients as they're currently being used in cosmetics. Still, it's hard to remove the taint of being associated with cancer, and not surprisingly, consumers are looking for alternatives. Enterprising raw material suppliers are eager to meet this emerging market. Case in point: this new organic preservative that Kaitlin asked about.

What is Arobocide?

Arobocide is an innovative ingredient from Active Micro Technologies (AMT) which is based on Leuconostoc spp. It is derived from a fermentation filtrate and contains non-viable microorganisms that can inhibit the growth of "bad" bacteria. Interesting fact: Leuconostoc spp is related to the micro-organisms used to create Kimchii, Korean fermented cabbage. It's a classic "No" product: No Ethoxylation, No Irradiation, No Sulphonation, No Ethylene Oxide treatment, No Hydrogenation and it's GMO Free. So, as far as we know, it has an excellent safety profile. But is it effective?

Does Arobocide work?
According to AMT's published data, Arobocide was tested against a variety of organisms, but they all appear to be a gram positive or negative. There's no indication this material is efficacious against molds and fungi. Broad spectrum protection is very important for cosmetic products. A preservative system that only protects against some microorganisms leaves the product vulnerable to contamination.

Also, we noticed that this material must be used at 2% to 4%, which is extraordinarily high for a preservative. Usually, these are used at a few tenths of a percent. We don't know the cost of this material, but it may be affordable only in the most high end of products. Finally, it's interesting that it apparently has some skin conditioning properties, so perhaps you can lower the level of other emollient ingredients to offset some of the cost.

THE BOTTOM LINE
It looks like this ingredient could be a safe choice if you're concerned about "chemical" preservatives. However, it does not have the broad spectrum activity required to effectively protect cosmetic products. So please be cautious if you choose to use this in products of your own or purchase products that use this as a preservative.

4 reasons why creating natural products is so hard

We're often asked why there aren't more truly natural products on the market. Here are the reasons why, from a cosmetic chemist's perspective.

Natural formulating is hard

First, formulating natural is hard. This is because the cosmetic products that currently exist are pretty good. Most people are satisfied with the performance of their skin creams and hair products. They are always seeking new products, but for the most part, cosmetics work as described. This has created a certain expectation of performance in the consumer's mind for any product they will buy. If you sell a product that does not perform as well as one that the consumer is used to, they will not continue to buy your product. Unfortunately, when you limit yourself to only "natural" ingredients, you cut out a lot of the best-performing ingredients. You reduce the number of surfactants you can use, the polymers, the preservatives, the fragrances and more. It is like being a painter and trying to use 3 colors versus competitors who can use 300. It is hard!

There is no standard definition

Another problem of natural formulating is that there are no standard definitions. There are a few different systems and we've written about natural formulating standards (http://thebeautybrains.com/tHgpm) before. But there is not yet a requirement for any company to follow those standards. If you wanted to create your own all-natural cosmetic line you would have to compete with companies who produce pseudo-natural cosmetic lines which are produced using standard ingredients with natural ingredients sprinkled in. These products will work better than yours. You would be at a marketing disadvantage. But that is the challenge of natural formulating.

Safety

One of the biggest challenges of natural formulating is that your products have to be proven safe. It is illegal to sell unsafe cosmetics in the United States and elsewhere in the world. Since most of the ingredients that you would use in cosmetics are capable of being contaminated with microbial growth, you will have to use some kind of preservative to prevent that. Unfortunately, the ingredients that are really effective at killing disease-causing microbes are not natural. You are severely limited in the ingredients you can use. This means that unless you have some special air-tight packaging made under anti-septic conditions or you have an expiration date on your product, you will not be able to honestly create an all-natural, preservative free cosmetic formulation. We know there are companies out there that claim they are, but most are using tricks to pretend they are not using preservatives when they actually are. This is an extremely difficult problem.

Performance
As we said before, formulating natural products is hard, and you have to face the fact that the best formulated cosmetic product is not going to work as well as the best formulated cosmetic product which is not restricted to only natural ingredients. And consumers buy cosmetics for their functionality. Yes, they say they want natural and organic. They say it makes them feel better about their purchases. But when it comes down to it, for most consumers, if your product does not perform as well as one of the pseudo-natural formulations, they will not continue to buy your product.

Why natural?
Considering the disadvantages that you are going to face in creating natural products, you have to ask yourself, why formulate natural at all? The reality is that naturally formulated cosmetic products are not more safe than standard cosmetic products. You may disagree with that, but your disagreement is not based on any kind of science or testing. Cosmetics have been safety tested and have proven to be some of the safest consumer products that anyone can buy. By restricting yourself to ingredients that are arbitrarily considered "natural", you are not making them automatically more safe. In fact,

there is evidence that unprocessed, natural ingredients are sometimes less safe due to bacterial and microbial contamination.

THE BOTTOM LINE

So, be sure to ask yourself why you want to formulate (or buy) naturally. You may still want to because it has proven to be a profitable marketing angle. Unfortunately, it is not a good formulating angle. Ultimately, consumers will buy products that are effective. Whether they are considered "natural" or not is just a bonus.

Skin care/makeup questions

Is vegan nail lacquer any good?

Lana says...I'm thinking of getting OCC's Nail Lacquer because it's vegan. How do they make it vegan? Will it be as good as a regular polish?

According to OCC's website, their products are vegan because they don't contain "animal-derived ingredients (including lanolin, beeswax, carmine and more)." We'll let you in on a little secret–it's not that hard to make a nail polish without these animal-derived ingredients.

Nail polishes don't contain many animal ingredients
Consider that nail polishes primarily consist of polymers, resins, and solvents. A few of these are derived from plant sources (ethyl alcohol can come from corn and stearic acid used in some esters comes from coconut oil, for example) but most of which are derived from petroleum.

WHAT? A vegan product contains synthetic petrochemicals? Yep!

OCC Vegan Nail Lacquer Ingredients
Ethyl Acetate, N-Butyl Acetate, Nitrocellulose, Isopropyl Alcohol, N-Butyl Alcohol, Styrene/Acryates Copolymer, Stearalkonium Hectorite, Benzophenone | May Contain: Iron Oxides, Titanium Dioxide, Ultramarines, Bismuth Oxychloride, FD&C Yellow #5, D&C Red #7, D&C Red #34, Ferric Ferrocyanine, Mica

THE BOTTOM LINE
Bully for them for taking a stance in favor of defenseless animals. But to be honest, this vegan product is not much different than a regular, animal-hating nail polish. But hey, they're not charging you that much more for this brand, so as long as you like their colors (our personal favorite is called "Captain Howdy") , then go for it. However, beware of any nail polish that wants you to pay more for the privilege of being "vegan."

Is DIY mascara safe?

Nancy says...Beautylish has recipes for DIY mascara. Not sure if this sounds hygienic. Does it put you at risk of getting an eye infection?

I guess this is as close as we get to providing a public service announcement: Do not use homemade mascara!

DIY Danger

Beautylish (http://thebeautybrains.com/EbkXE), the site referenced by Nancy, recommends making your own mascara by mixing aloe vera gel with powdered charcoal. Supposedly, the benefit of this approach is that you avoid preservatives and "excess chemicals." Unfortunately, whoever wrote this post is not very well informed about cosmetic science and is actually advocating something that is MORE dangerous, not less. Here is what we would say to the writer of that post:

Aloe Vera gel is not preservative free

First, if your goal is to create a safer product by avoiding preservatives then you've failed from the start because aloe vera gel HAS preservatives in it. Depending on the manufacturer, aloe vera gel can be preserved by a combination of sodium benzoate, sodium sulphate, potassium sorbate, and ascorbic acid. But wait, it gets worse: not only are you using preservatives, but you're using the WRONG ones. We couldn't find any mascaras that use these as preservatives. You should use preservatives which have been tested and shown to safe for use around the eye, such as Imidazolidinyl Urea, Methylparaben, Propylparaben, and Phenoxyethanol. You're creating a formula that may grow dangerous bacteria.

Colorants for eyes need to be tested

Second, the activated charcoal you're using is not approved as a colorant for use around the eye. The FDA requires that each batch of colorants used around the eye are certified, and that they comply with safety regulations. A jar of activated charcoal won't have that safety assurance. Who knows what kind of contaminants it may contain?

THE BOTTOM LINE

Ask which you think is safer: Purchasing a professionally formulated product with ingredients that have been shown to be safe for use around the eye and that have been tested to ensure it won't support growth of bacteria that could potentially lead to dangerous eye infection, OR mixing two ingredients, one of which is not properly preserved and the other which is not designed to be used close to your eyes? (Whew, pardon the run on sentence!)

We're sorry, but you couldn't pay us enough to risk an eye infection by "protecting" ourselves from excess chemicals.

Is Aloe Vera really chemical free?

Gina asks...I need a clarification on this botanical. I know that there are these natural forms of aloe barbadensis. But what is aloe barbadensis gel? Is it all-natural or is it made of one of the other forms by the help of some chemical?

Ah, the vagaries of cosmetic ingredient nomenclature. Here are the officially recognized terms for different versions of Aloe Barbadensis.

• Aloe vera identification

• Aloe barbadensis flower extract

• Aloe barbadensis leaf extract

• Aloe barbadensis leaf juice

• Aloe barbadensis leaf juice powder

• Aloe barbadensis leaf polysaccharides

• Aloe barbadensis leaf water

As you can see, "aloe barbadensis gel" is not on the list, and so it's not an officially recognized name for aloe vera. So, suppliers can use the "gel" name as long as their Material Safety Data Sheet uses one of the official names. For example, one supplier sells aloe barbadensis gel and lists the the following as the "real" names:

• EU Substance Name: Aloe vera extract

• EU INCI Name: Aloe barbadensis Leaf Extract

• CTFA INCI Name: Aloe barbadensis Leaf Juice

• JCIA INCI Name: Aloe barbadensis Leaf Extract

So the answer to your first question is sort of "all of the above."

Are there chemicals in my aloe vera?
To answer your second question, we have to look at what ingredients are added to the "aloe." If you buy any kind of water containing aloe

216

extract, it will also contain some kind of preservative. For example, one supplier uses a combination of sodium benzoate, sodium sulphate, potassium sorbate, and ascorbic acid to preserve their aloe barbadensis leaf extract.

THE BOTTOM LINE
There can be hidden "extras" in ingredients that appear to be all natural.

Is this lip balm unique?

Penny ponders....I am wondering what makes this YuBe lip balm unique and if it is worth more or more effective than the brands I normally buy at Wal-Mart.

We're not sure which brand you normally use, but let's compare YuBe with a couple of other popular lip balms, Burt's Bees and Chapstick.

How are YuBe ingredients different?

The YuBe product is made entirely of plant derived ingredients. Burt's Bees balm is similar, except that it uses carmine (from insects) and fragrance (which could be synthetic). Both use beeswax as the primary stiffening agent. The Chapstick product uses some petroleum based ingredients (petrolatum, etc) and some animal derived ingredients (lanolin compounds). It uses a plant wax (carnauba) as the main stiffening agent. All three products will make your lips feel good, but if plant-sourced ingredients are a must have for you, then you'll want to stick with YuBe or Burt's Bees.

Is YuBE a good value?

Of course, you'll pay more for the privilege of saving the environment from the evils of petrochemicals:

YuBe: $5.00/stick

Burts Bees: $3.00/stick.

Chapstick: $1.25/ stick.

YuBe ingredients

Glycine Soja (Soybean) Oil, Cera Alba (Beeswax), Prunus Amygdalus Dulcis (Sweet Almond) Oil, Butyrospermum Parkii (Shea Butter) Fruit, Cocos Nucifera (Coconut) Oil, Camphor, Tocopherol (Vitamin E), Aloe Barbadensis (Aloe Vera), Eupato-rium Rebaudianum Bertoni (Stevia) Leaf Extract, Rosmarinus Officinalis (Rosemary Leaf Extract).

Burt's Bees ingredients

Helianthus Annuus (Sunflower) Seed Oil, Beeswax (Apis Mellifera), Cocos Nucifera (Coconut) Oil, Castor (Ricinus Communis) Seed Oil, Lanolin, Comfrey (Symphytum Officinale) Root Extract, Pomegranate Oil, Prunus Amygdalus Dulcis (Sweet Almond) Oil, Anise Oil, Cassia Oil, Cinnamon Leaf Oil, Clary Sage (Salvia Sclarea) Oil, Citrus Reticulata (Mandarin) Oil, Tocopheryl Acetate (Vitamin E), Rosmarinus Officinalis (Rosemary) Extract, Carmine (CI 75470), Fragrance

Chapstick ingredients

Active Ingredients: Padimate (1.5%), White Petrolatum (44%)

Inactive Ingredients: Arachidyl Propionate, Camphor, Carnauba (Copernicia Cerifera) Wax, Cetearyl Alcohol, D&C Red 6 Barium Lake (CI 15850), Fragrance, Isopropyl Lanolate, Isopropyl Myristate, Lanolin, Lemon (Citrus Medica Limonium) Oil, Light Mineral Oil, Maltol, Methylparaben, Octyldodecanol, Beeswax (Apis Mellifera), Phenyltrimethicone, Propylparaben, Saccharin, White Wax

THE BOTTOM LINE

If you like the feel provided by naturals oils and waxes, and you can afford the upcharge, then YuBe may be for you. But there's nothing unique about the formula that makes it work better than cheaper lip balms.

New natural acne cure

The Beauty Brains are often accused of unfairly bashing natural products. Typically this bashing is accompanied by an additional accusation that we're "paid off" by the Big Chemical Companies so they can keep on selling nasty chemical products instead of safer and cheaper natural alternatives. To be honest, nothing is farther from the truth. Whenever we find evidence-based reasons to believe in natural remedies, we promote those solutions just as we would any "synthetic chemical."

Time for Thyme

Case in point: The Dermatology Times reported on a study out of Leeds University in England. The researchers tested several natural extracts for efficacy in killing p. acnes, the bacteria that contributes to the formation of zits. They found that a tincture of thyme was not only more effective than the other natural extracts tested, but was actually superior in efficacy to benzoyl peroxide, one of the approved drug ingredients. (BP, of course, is made by the Big Chemical Companies.) In addition, since the thyme tincture is less irritating than benzyl peroxide, it's likely to result in increased usage. The power of this herb doesn't really surprise us, since we've always been told that "thyme heals all wounds." (Sorry, we couldn't resist.)

THE BOTTOM LINE

Of course, more research needs to be done. The presence or absence of this bacteria is only one of the triggering mechanisms for acne. Still, it's very promising when a natural ingredient shows true efficacy. We're just worried what will happen when the Big Chemical Companies find out that we've broken this story. Maybe we should re-watch the movie Silkwood.

What is cupuacu?

Connie asks... What can you tell us about Cupuacu and the best place to buy it?

Cupuacu is a tropical fruit (or is it a nut?) that is similar to the cacao nut (or is it fruit?) According to those in the know, Cupauacu smells like a cross between chocolate and pineapple and tastes like pear mixed with banana. The pulp is rich in fatty materials (similar to cocoa butter) that make it an excellent moisturizer. In addition, research has shown that the seeds contain no less than nine known antioxidants (warning: this list of chemical names may make your head spin just a little bit):

> "(+)-catechin, (-)-epicatechin, isoscutellarein 8-O-beta-d-glucuronide, hypolaetin 8-O-beta-d-glucuronide, quercetin 3-O-beta-d-glucuronide, quercetin 3-O-beta-d-glucuronide 6 '-methyl ester, quercetin, kaempferol, and isoscutellarein 8-O-beta-d-glucuronide 6 '-methyl ester."

THE BOTTOM LINE

Cupuacu is another natural ingredient that may have beneficial properties. Unfortunately, as we've previously reported, it's difficult to access the effect of antioxidants on skin, so it's unclear whether or not all these phyto-chemicals really provide an additional benefit. Still, this stuff smells great, and it's a great moisturizer, so there seems little downside in trying it. (Assuming, of course that there are no ethical sourcing issues – you know how sensitive our rainforests are!)

Does pressed powder makeup always contain synthetic ingredients?

Mia asks... Is it possible to make pressed makeup without using any synthetics?

Rather than re-opening the debate on natural vs synthetic, we'll try to address your question as it applies specifically to powdered makeup.

Loose powder needs fewer ingredients
One can certainly make the case that certain brands of so-called mineral makeup are among the most "natural" of cosmetic products. For example, Mineral Hygenics only contains a few powders which are all derived from crushed rocks (more or less). This kind of product is relatively easy to formulate using only mineral (i.e., "natural") ingredients, because it's just a simple blend of powders.

Pressed powder is more complex
Pressed powders, on the other hand, are much more complex. In order for the powders to stay compressed, they need some kind of binding oil. And for those oils to mix with the powders, they may require a surfactant to lower the surface tension. And the pressed powders have to spread easily across your skin, so they may require emollients to provide slip. And these surfactants and binders and emollients may require antioxidants to prevent rancidity. And, since pressed powders have a surface that comes in contact with fingers and makeup brushes, they are more likely to require preservatives than loose powders. AND...well you get the idea.

The more ingredients that a formula requires, the more difficult it becomes to source ingredients that everyone will agree are "natural." And although natural alternatives may be available, they may not work as well as the nasty old "synthetic" chemicals. This is particularly true of preservatives and of many surfactants.

THE BOTTOM LINE

It's not impossible to formulate a pressed powder without "synthetics", but the requirements of the formula make it much more difficult. If you're allergic to specific ingredients, it may be worthwhile to switch to a pressed powder. But if you're just afraid of "synthetics", you needn't worry.

Is 100% natural lipstick worth the hype?

Brenda asks...Since I've been trying to get pregnant over the last year, I've become more concerned about toxicity. I probably eat a sizable amount of lipstick. I am not your usual "organic" type, but I was surprised to see the list of ingredients for my favorite lipstick, Avon's Beyond Color Plumping Lipstick. Are organic lipsticks worth the hype? I've seen that Bare Minerals has a natural lipstick, but I'm not feeling $25 per tube. I'm more of a drugstore type girl. I'm not loaded with money and don't want to be more paranoid than I should be.

"Regular" lipstick like the Avon example you gave costs $8.00 ($3.99 on sale!) where as the Bare Minerals "100% natural" lipstick is $25. It's really impossible for us to make the value judgment for you, but we can help by telling you if there are any significant technical differences between the two. (One point of clarification: although you asked about Bare Minerals "organic" lipstick, the company does not make the claim that this product is organic. They only state that it is "100% natural".)

Ingredient comparison
It looks like the Bare Minerals formula is quite different from a typical lipstick, because a) it only uses iron oxide pigments as colorants, and b) it does not contain any of the petroleum-derived emollients typically found in lipsticks.

Natural vs synthetic
As you're probably aware, the debate over the safety of natural versus synthetic ingredients is not as simple as "all natural is good and all synthetic is bad." For example, synthetic dyes, like those used in the Avon product, are accused of containing carcinogens. And natural lavender extract, like the oil used in the Bare Minerals lipstick, is said to cause headaches and irritate skin. Whether or not you believe any of these specific accusations is beside the point, but it's important to recognize that these ingredients are ALL chemicals and depending on the dose, chemicals may have undesirable side effects.

So rather than make this a debate about toxicology, we'll try to answer your question by making a couple of quick assumptions to simplify the argument about whether an ingredient is "natural" or not. This is no trivial point, since currently there is no standard definition for "natural" as it relates to beauty products. But for the sake of this discussion, we rated each product based on four basic factors as described below:

Compromises in lip colors
Contains only "mineral colorants" (no synthetic dyes)

Avon: No

Bare Minerals: Yes

Contains only mineral or plant derived waxes and emollients
Avon: No

Bare Minerals: Yes

Provides long lasting color
Avon: Yes

Bare Minerals: No

Offers a wide range of colors
Avon: Yes

Bare Minerals: No

These four factors demonstrate the tradeoffs that you typically have to make when choosing natural products: if you want to avoid "synthetic" chemicals, you'll have to accept a limited number of color choices. (That's because iron oxides, the mineral pigments used to provide color, are only available in a few reddish-brownish-yellowish shades.) You'll also have to give up long lasting color, because these iron oxides don't stain lips like synthetic dyes do. Are these good trade-offs to make? Maybe, but we can't make that value judgment for you. We can only try to frame the question and provide a few helpful facts.

THE BOTTOM LINE

Unfortunately, there is no easy, one-size-fits-all answer to your question. Whether or not so-called natural lipstick is a good value depends on what's most important to you. If you want to limit potential intake of "chemicals" (even though the best science available doesn't indicate that this is a significant risk) AND if you don't mind a limited number of "earth-tone" colors, then a "100% Natural" product may be a good choice for you. But you'll need to spend more for those benefits.

Is Astaxanthin a good natural sunscreen?

Jemma asks...I actually saw that Eve Pearl uses astaxanthin in her makeup, which is meant to be a natural sunscreen. Apparently it doesn't make you look whitish like other sunscreens and, being a super antioxidant, its great for the skin. I want to try buying a few caps and mixing them in my makeup, but apparently its highly orange in color. Do you have any knowledge about astaxanthin?

Astaxanthin has been a hot topic ever since the article in the Huffington post that suggests recapping research suggesting it could be a "sunscreen pill." (We're not sure, but we think Astaxanthin was also a character on "Xena Warrior Princess.") Anyway, it looks like it may have the potential to help protect the body against free radicals. However, that's much different than what you're asking about here, Jasmine. That's because the mode of action of a free radical suppressant, which is ingested, is going to be much different than a UV absorber, which is applied topically. So will smearing astaxanthin on our skin help protect us against the damaging rays of the sun?

Two reasons why astaxanthin is not a good sun screen
The first hurdle to overcome before a chemical can be a good UV absorber is that it has to be able to absorb UV rays. This sounds obvious, but if it can't absorb light in the right region of the spectrum, then it's a nonstarter as far as being a sunscreen is concerned.

If you visit our Forum (http://thebeautybrains.com/eRZQa), you'll see a couple of graphs showing how astaxanthin absorbs light. As you'll see, it absorbs visible rays very strongly, but it hardly absorbs UV rays at all. In other words, it's pretty much useless as a sunscreen.

Not that you need another reason, but since we promised you two, here you go: astaxanthin also has a characteristic carrot-like orange color. (It's related to carotene.) It reminds us of some of the early sunless tanner formulations that gave the skin a ghastly orange hue. Even if it absorbed properly, the aesthetics of this ingredient would limit its use. Also the final nail in the coffin is that this ingredient is expensive and would be cost prohibitive in regular sunscreen formulas.

THE BOTTOM LINE
While we're anxiously watching future research on internal sunscreens, this ingredient will not make Eve Pearl's lotion work any better, so don't waste your money.

How does witch hazel work?

Linda says...How do tannins found in witch hazel act as an astringent? And how is witch hazel modified from its original state to its state in cosmetics?

After reading the StevenFoster educational monograph (http:// thebeautybrains.com/L8EAC) we're now equipped to tell you more than you ever wanted to know about witch hazel.

How does witch hazel act as an astringent?

First, we'll explain that astringents are materials that give the skin a feeling of tightness. In the case of witch hazel the active ingredient is a chemical called a tannin. (At the time of this writing it's close to Christmas, so we're tempted to work in some kind of pun about a "tannin bomb." But we won't.) Anyway, tannins can cross link proteins, causing biological structures like skin to literally "tighten up." (Note: sometimes alcohol evaporation can give this impression.)

How is witch hazel modified from its original form?

In its natural form, witch hazel is a shrub that can grow to be 10 or more feet tall. It has oval leaves and slender petals. In autumn, the plant is harvested by cutting the branches to the ground and chipping the wood and leaves into little bite size pieces. This mulch is then transferred to large stainless-steel vats, where it is steam distilled for thirty-six hours. After "stewing", the extracted mixture is condensed and filtered, and ethanol is added as a preservative. (Depending on the exact processing, the witch hazel may contain more or less tannins. The mixture of plant parts also controls the tannin content – bark contains 31 times more tannin than the leaves.) The resulting liquid is bottled and sold to drug stores as "witch hazel."

THE BOTTOM LINE

When it comes to "natural" ingredients, witch hazel is about as natural as it gets. However, it's questionable whether or not the skin tightening effect it provides really has any benefit for skin. Certainly all the alcohol it contains can be drying!

Why are Clean and Clear oil absorbing sheets made with mineral oil?

Marilyn must know...I remember using Clean & Clear oil absorbing sheets a few years ago, and I wanted to try them out again. However, I read the ingredients, and I noticed it had mineral oil. What is the purpose of the mineral oil, and do I need to be worried about using these on my oily skin?

Great question, Marilyn! Why in the world would an oil absorbing sheet contain oil? To get the answer we have to take a look at the ingredients.

Clean & Clear ingredients
Polypropylene

This is the plastic material used to create the sheets.

DMDBS

Also known as 3, 4 Dimethylbenzyl Idene Sorbitol, this is a modifier added to the melted polypropylene to form a complex nanofabril structure that gives the sheets their characteristic flexibility and helps "wick" oil away from the skin.

Mineral oil

This is a modifier for the plastic that reduces the cycle time for shaping and processing the sheets. It's also conceivable (although this is just a theory on our part), that the mineral oil in the plastic matrix may help with oil absorption, due to the chemical principle of "like dissolves like" (that's for all you hard core chemistry geeks in the audience).

Zinc stearate

Opacifier that makes the sheets look creamy, not clear.

Ultramarines

Pigments which give the sheets their characteristic baby blue color.

THE BOTTOM LINE

Clean & Clear Oil absorbing sheets are a great way to degrease your face. The mineral oil used in their production is part of the plastic sheets themselves, so it won't make your oily skin any worse.

Hair care questions

How can I tell if my shampoo is really all natural?

Hanna asks...I actually bought a Rustic Art shampoo that claims to be all natural, does not test on animals, is pH balanced, contains no sulphates, is great for the environment and all those good things. I was skeptical, as I thought since it's so good it won't lather and might just clean my hair and won't be like using silicones and stuff...I didn't mind as I wanted a natural shampoo. To my surprise, it lathered really well...just needed a small amount too for the lather! Also my hair felt real soft by the end of the wash, which I never felt from other shampoos till I used a conditioner...I am really hooked to this and now I am skeptical if this is really using all natural ingredients

The trouble with answering a question such as this one is that there is no standard definition of "natural" for beauty products. But we'll see what we can do based on looking at the ingredients.

Rustic Art shampoo ingredients
Demineralized water, Cocamidopropyl Betaine (coconut oil extract), Ascorbic acid, Disodium cocoamphodiacetate, Hydrolised Wheat protein, Aloe Vera Juice, Sodium Cocoyl (?) essential oil Blend/Herbal oil blend, and AOS,a plant derivative used as surfactant.

Note: the ingredient list we were provided is not complete, as it uses partial names and abbreviations.

To make our point of how confusing the question of "natural" is, let's look at this through the lens of two different definitions and see how the answer changes.

Definition #1: A product is "all natural" if all ingredients are from renewable, non-petroleum resources.
Through this lens, this product would be rated very natural, because all of the ingredients can be derived from non-petroleum sources. For example, the surfactants are coconut-based and can be derived from

coconut oil. Ascorbic acid can be derived from fruit. The wheat derivative obviously comes from wheat, and so on. Based on this definition, this product does seem "all natural." So, if you like the answer from this definition, you should just stop reading here.

Definition # 2: A product is "all natural" if all ingredients are from renewable, non-petroleum resources AND all chemicals used in the processing of the main ingredients follow the same rule.
Hmmm. This is where it gets tricky. Let's look at the main ingredient in the formula, cocoamidopropyl betaine (CAPB), as an example. While coconut oil is a nice natural source for the backbone of this ingredient, several "non-natural" chemicals like chloroacetic acid must be used to transform the nutty oil into CAPB.

So you see the rabbit hole one jumps down when trying to pin down the definition of natural. Is it okay if there is only one non-natural ingredient used to form the product? What about two or three ingredients? What if one of those "unnatural ingredients" is very toxic or damaging to the environment – does that count against the natural-ness of the product? Or does it not matter since the backbone is coconut oil? There is no single right answer for these questions, so everyone is left to fend for themselves when it comes to natural definitions. Therefore, using Definition #2, one would be hard-pressed to describe this product as all natural.

It gets even more complicated when you start to layer in other factors, such as animal testing, biodegradability of ingredients, waste water management, sustainability (remember palm oil) and so on. So now you see how this works. Depending on the parameters of your natural definition, you can declare that everything is all natural, nothing is all natural, or it's somewhere in between.

THE BOTTOM LINE
Is this product all natural? If you're cool with Definition #1 and you like the way this makes your hair feel, then we'd say yes.

Is silk good for hair and skin?

Sandy says...Could you please explain the benefits and structure of using real silk byproducts in hair and skin care? ....And what might a substitute be?

If popularity is any indication of efficacy, then silk must really kick butt, because there are 42 different silk-based ingredients that are used in well over 1000 different beauty products (according to SkinDeep.) If only it really was a popularity contest.

Silk on hair
Silk protein is widely used in hair care formulations as a supplemental conditioning agent. If it's properly derivatized (i.e., chemically modified so it sticks to hair), we've seen evidence that it can help repair damage. (It can protect hair from exposure to alkaline processing such as you'd encounter during hair coloring or relaxing.)

Presumably, it works because of its ability to form a protective film on hair. There's plenty of research by the raw material manufacturers that silk has conditioning benefits when delivered from the right vehicle, but it's impossible to tell which finished goods manufacturers are using the silk at the required levels to deliver that benefit.

Sadly, in most hair products, silk protein in all its various forms is only used at token amounts to provide a label claim. The rest of the ingredients in the formula are much more impactful in terms of providing conditioning benefits.

Silk on skin
Since skin, unlike hair, is a living organ, we're always hopeful that certain ingredients may be able to provide more of a beneficial effect. In the case of silk, we were able to find one reference (http://thebeautybrains.com/fEnbm) that indicates a specific type of silk (Sericin from the middle silk gland of the Bombyx mori silkworm) has antioxidant properties that are beneficial to skin. It can also inhibit lipid per oxidation and is able to reduce UVB-induced symp-

toms in both short and long term treatments. Interestingly, it can also chelate with copper.

Once again, however, the challenge is to know which products contain the right kind of silk at efficacious levels. That's difficult, if not impossible, to ascertain without detailed information from the manufacturer. Looking at the list of ingredients can be directionally helpful, but there's no way to tell for sure how much of a given ingredient is present. If the company is using patented technology, there may be a patent disclosure which reveals how much silky goodness the product contains.

THE BOTTOM LINE
Despite its popularity, for the most part, silk is used as a "feel good" ingredient in cosmetic products. There is some research that it can protect skin from UV damage, which makes us hopeful that someone will market an efficacious silk-based product.

Can vinegar remove minerals from hair?

Mindy asks...How about just rinsing hair with a vinegar/water rinse [to remove mineral buildup]? I use vinegar to remove the buildup of minerals elsewhere; wouldn't it do the same on my hair?

Many shampoos claim to remove minerals with chelating agents that can bind the minerals. But what about an acid rinse, as Marcia suggests? Surely vinegar can't work as well as a product specially formulated to remove minerals, can it? The answer surprised even us!

We decided to test the hypothesis for ourselves. Since it's hard to see mineral deposits on hair, we used the next best thing – a shower faucet. Weeks of exposure to relatively hard shower water had dulled the shiny metal faucet with an easily visible mineral residue. (You can see the actual pictures here on our blog: http://the beautybrains.com/nPQ4C.)

Vinegar vs Water
For the first part of the test, we wiped the left side of the faucet with a paper towel dampened with regular kitchen vinegar and the right side with plain water. The vinegar removes significantly more mineral buildup than water alone.

Vinegar vs Chelator
Next, we decided to see how well vinegar would do against a product designed for removing buildup: Tilex Tub and Tile Cleaner. Once again, we used vinegar on the left with the cleaning product on the right. Surprisingly, the vinegar works about as well as the specially designed cleanser!

THE BOTTOM LINE
While this is more of a demonstration than an actual experiment to prove that vinegar removes minerals from hair, it is certainly encouraging enough to give it a try. And vinegar is certainly more "green" (and cheaper) than chelating shampoo!

Is apple cider vinegar really good for hair?

Skippy says...I have started incorporated Apple Cider Vinegar (ACV) rinses in my hair care practices with great results. My hair is very, very kinky and I find if I do the apple cider vinegar rinse as the final cleaning step of washing my hair, my hair feels smoother, reflects light more (shinier) and it is easier to detangle. But what is the apple cider vinegar really doing to my hair?

In actual lab testing, we've haven't been able to demonstrate much of an effect from vinegar. But since vinegar is an acid, in theory, there are three things that the low pH could be doing for your hair.

Three Ways That Apple Cider Vinegar May Help Hair

1. Tightening the cuticle.

If your hair is damaged and the cuticles are upraised, an acid rinse could be helping them to lay flatter and therefore improving shine and detangle-ability.

2. Boosting conditioner efficacy

Conditioners based on quaternary ammonium compounds work better at a lower pH because they stick to hair better. Maybe the vinegar is helping to "lock" your conditioner onto the hair.

3. Removing shampoo residue

If shampoo isn't rinsed completely, it can leave a dulling residue on hair. Vinegar may be helping to remove buildup and letting the natural hair shine through.

THE BOTTOM LINE

Again, these are only theories. We have no proof that ACV is really good for your hair. The general scientific consensus is that condition-er will do a much better job than any kind of vinegar rinse. However, if you find that it works well for your hair, there's really no downside to using it.

Are there any natural hair color products?

Mary Ellen asks...Do you know of any natural hair color product on the market yet (other than Henna) for people to use in place of the ones on the market with harsh chemicals? I've heard of a few salons that have options for consumers, but they don't allow us to purchase them and use on our own. It seems there is a trend right now in the beauty industry with natural ingredients, and I'm wondering if you've heard of anyone coming up with hair color that regular consumers can buy and that actually works without too much complication.

We've got good news and bad news for you. The good news is that this is a very easy question to answer. The bad news is you're not going to like the answer!

Chemical colorants

There are a number of natural materials that can stain hair. Henna, as you mentioned in your question, is one. Certain fruit and berry extracts also work well in this regard (especially if you're looking for a nice strawberry red or blueberry blue).

But if you're looking for the shades that are traditionally associated with permanent hair color, there is no "natural" solution at this time. Part of the reason for this is that no staining material can lighten hair. The natural melanin pigment in dark hair must be destroyed in order to make hair lighter, and this requires a fairly strong chemical reaction.

THE BOTTOM LINE

If you're concerned about synthetic chemicals, you should be very skeptical of any "natural" hair dyes, because there is NO natural way to truly color hair.

Can honey lighten hair?

PL says…There's a video on Youtube by Andrea's Choice. She used honey to lighten up her hair. I haven't tried but you can watch the video.

Thanks, PL, for the link to this video (http://thebeautybrains.com /zovkl) where Andrea explains how mixing honey (either raw or regular) with either olive oil and banana or with just your regular conditioner can lighten hair. She claims the honey contains peroxide that can bleach hair over time. But does this really work?

Hair lightening science
It's true that honey contains peroxide. (http://thebeautybrains.com /I9jNQ) More accurately, it contains an enzyme, glucose oxidase, that can produce peroxide. But keep in mind that peroxide is only an effective bleaching agent at the right concentration and at the right pH.

Concentration: how much peroxide is in honey?
How much peroxide do you need to lighten hair? To fully bleach hair, it takes a solution of peroxide at a concentration of 6%; 3% can be used over time to gradually lighten hair. Glucose oxidase in honey can react to release peroxide under the right conditions. (It's also important to note that only raw honey contains this active enzyme.) When honey is diluted with water, the enzyme can produce about 1 milimole of peroxide per liter, which is about 1000 times less than the 3% solution required to bleach hair. This is far too little to have a significant effect on your hair.

Okay, but just for the sake of argument, let's say that you used a LOT of honey on your hair. Would it work then? Only if the pH was right.

The pH required for bleaching hair
Peroxide solutions must be "activated" by increasing the pH, because peroxide is not very reactive at any pH below 4. Typically, peroxide is mixed with ammonia, because it has a very high pH. The pH of honey

is between 3.2 and 4.5, which is far below the range required for effective hair bleaching.

What about Andrea's tip about mixing honey with conditioner? Would that make it work better? Well, the pH of conditioner is in the 4-5 range (conditioners work better on the acid side, because they protonate or increase the positive charge of the goodies that stick to your hair.) So even mixed with conditioner the pH is still too low be effective.

THE BOTTOM LINE
If you use the right kind of honey and if the enzyme is still active and if you dilute it properly and if you adjust it to the right pH and IF you get it on your hair before it's used up by reaction with the rest of the organic stuff in the mixture, then you'll STILL have only about 1/1000 of the amount you need to lighten your hair. Just because Winnie the Pooh was blonde doesn't mean that honey can lighten your hair.

Is grape seed oil good for protecting hair from heat?

Tina asks...I'm transitioning from relaxed to natural hair, and a lot of blogs and video bloggers tout grape seed oil as a heat protectant when blowdrying or flat ironing hair, because it has a high smoke point (about 420 °F). Is there any truth to this claim? The smoke point refers to the oil's use in cooking, but does it apply to hair as well?

When it comes to protecting hair from heat damage, there's more to it than just how much heat the ingredients can take.

What to look for in a good heat protectant
Heat tolerance (in this case measured by smoke point of the oil) is only one factor to consider. You also need to look at how the product lubricates hair. You can experiment with oils if you want DIY heat protection, but be careful: oils alone can create drag which could slow down the flat iron as it passes through your hair, so it could end up doing MORE damage.

Good heat protectants should also help offset the drying effects of heat. Ideally, you want a combination of glycerine or other moisturizers to lock in water and a low molecular weight polymer that can penetrate and help prevent heat from cracking the cuticles.

Which oils can stand a lot of heat
But back to your question about smoke point. The reference that we found lists the smoke point of grape seed at 485F, soy bean oil at 495F, safflower oil at 510F, and avocado oil at a startling 520F! Wikipedia lists slightly different values: Cottonseed and virgin olive oil are in the same range as grape seed while almond, peanut, sunflower, and our cold friend coconut oil are higher. We're not sure which values are more accurate, but either way it looks like you have some options to try that offer an even higher smoke point than grape seeds.

THE BOTTOM LINE

Feel free to experiment with different oils, but be careful that you don't damage your hair in the process. While it may not be as "green", you could also try a good heat protectant leave in conditioner.

Is amla powder good for hair?

Amy asks...What is Amla powder and what does it do for hair?

Amla, also known as Indian gooseberry, is a fruit from the myrobalan-tree, which is native to India and Burma. Like its cousin, the North American gooseberry, amla fruit is edible with tart citrusy flavor. It's allegedly high in ascorbic acid (vitamin C) and tannins, which give it high antioxidant strength. Amla also contains flavonoids, kaempferol, ellagic acid and gallic acid.

Preliminary medical research has shown Amla potentially provides a surprising variety of benefits, including antiviral and antimicrobial properties, prevention of rheumatoid arthritis and osteoporosis, activity against some cancers, reduced severity of acute pancreatitis, age-related renal disease, and diabetes, and reduction of blood cholesterol levels. Not bad, eh?

Is Amla good for hair?

It's popularly believed that amla fruit is good for hair when applied as a conditioner. A quick search reveals claims about nourishing hair and scalp, adding texture and volume to hair, and preventing premature grey hair. Does amla really deliver against any of these claims?

"Nourishing" claims are fairly ambiguous and are therefore easy to support. Any material that provides a conditioning effect can be said to be nourishing, so it's likely that amla does have some benefit in this regard. Texturizing may be one area where amla really delivers, provided it's left in your hair. We've read a number of anecdotal stories of these benefits from people who've tried amla oil for hair.

The gray hair claims may come from the fact that amla is used in inks and fabric dyes to help "fix" the dye in place. Unfortunately, hair dyes work by a different chemistry than fabric dyes, and we can find no reference to in the cosmetic science literature to indicate that amla has any effect on hair color what so ever.

What about Amla Oil?

While Amy didn't specifically ask about it, amla fruit is also available in oil form. We would be very cautious about purchasing this version, because in several of the products we reviewed, the so-called "amla oil" was really just amla extract diluted down in mineral and canola oil. You're better off with the concentrated powder.

THE BOTTOM LINE

While some of the claims are outlandish, you may perceive some basic conditioning and texturizing benefits from applying amla powder to your hair. We'd expect this to be true of leave in applications and wouldn't expect to see any difference when it's rinsed out.

Interesting bonus fact: In Punjabi, amla is called olay, as in "Oil of Olay" beauty products from Proctor and Gamble. Is this coincidence, or sinister design?

Is beer good for your hair?

Brewski has a sobering question...I see a lot of conversation about beer rinse and heat damage; I was wondering if a Brain could shed some light on this?

Beer is a great way to treat heat damage; we always feel better after downing a couple of frosty beverages...Oh wait. You were asking about beer on HAIR. That's different. There are three reasons that beer MIGHT help protect your hair from heat damage. Do you think they could be true?

3 Reasons Beer Could Be Good For Hair
Beer contains protein, which can form a strengthening film on your hair.

Beer has an acidic pH, which makes your hair shiny by tightening the cuticles.

Beer contains hops, which are natural astringents.

The sobering truth
Beer contains grain proteins (like corn, wheat, or rice), but the protein is not chemically modified to deposit on your hair – it just rinses down the drain!

The low pH of beer is caused by dissolved carbon dioxide, which will not have a significant impact, because loose cuticles are caused by loss of the natural hair lipids that hold them in place.

It's true that hops have a mild astringent effect on skin, but they are in very low concentrations in beer and are not left on your hair long enough to have an effect anyway.

THE BOTTOM LINE
From a scientific perspective, putting beer on your hair is just a waste of good brew.

Can herbal extracts style hair?

Kitty's question...I'm considering getting a "Twist Defining Cream", and it has a bunch of extracts listed near the top of the list. Are they delivering the promise of the product, or are they just pixie dust?

The best way to answer this question it is to look at what the product is supposed to do and then assess whether the natural extracts in the formula help it perform that function or not.

Based on the ingredients that you gave us (which are listed below), we're guessing that this is the "As I Am" Twist cream. Here's what their website has to say about the product:

> "Shiny smoothness (and lots of it), is what you'll get when you twist with this one-of-a-kind rich creamy styler. Made especially for highly textured hair with nurturing natural oils, plus an organic extract that provides the ultimate in moisturization. There's even a wondrous organic compound blended in that works to block DHT and stimulate healthy hair growth."

So, to summarize, they are saying the three key functions of this product are to help:

• Give you a twisty style

• Smooth and moisturize hair

• Stimulate hair growth by blocking DHT.

As I Am Twist Defining Cream Ingredients
> *Aqueous (Water, Aqua Purificada, Purified) Extracts: Cocos Nucifera (Coconut)[1] and Phyllanthus Emblica (Amla)[1] and Citrus Reticulata (Tangerine)[1] and Beta Vulgaris (Beet) Root[1], Glycerin[1], Acetamide MEA, Helianthus Annuus (Sunflower) Seed Oil1, Ricinus Communis (Castor) Seed Oil[1], Triethanolamine, Cocos Nucifera (Coconut) Oil[1], Butyrospermum Parkii (Shea Butter)[1], Carbomer, Phytosterols[2], Disodium Ethylene Dicocamide PEG-15 Disulfate, Sodium Lauroyl Lactylate, Behenyl Alcohol[1], Glyc-*

eryl Stearate, Glyceryl Stearate Citrate, Trideceth-12, TBHQ, Diazolidinyl Urea, Iodopropynyl Butylcarbamate, Potassium Sorbate, Fragrance/Parfum, Limonene.

How plausible are their claims?

The last claim is the most outrageous. There are a lot of products that talk about blocking DHT, but there's no evidence that this is effective in restoring hair growth. If it were, it would be a drug product, so it doesn't matter whether the ingredients are botanicals or not.

The second claim is more plausible. Natural oils can be highly effective as smoothing and moisturizing agents, especially in a leave on product. Both coconut oil and shea butter are excellent refatting agents for hair, and we've blogged many times about how coconut oil can penetrate into the cortex and strengthen hair.

The first claim about hair styling is plausible, but doesn't require natural ingredients; it requires waxy materials or even styling polymers. Looking at the ingredient list, we see that the formula includes Sodium Lauroyl Lactylate, Behenyl Alcohol, and Glyceryl Stearate, which will help hold the hair in place because of their thick, waxy consistency. But even though these may be sourced from coconut oil, these are clearly not "botanical extracts."

It's a numbers game

You can also look at it this way: there are approximately 2 dozen ingredients in this formula. Of those ingredients, we'd say about eight of them are could be considered "botanical extracts." Of those, probably only five are contributing any functionality to the formula. We're being a bit generous here, because we're guessing the coconut and shea are doing most of the moisturizing and not the castor oil, sunflower oil or the amla.

THE BOTTOM LINE

We'd say that the botanical ingredients in this Twist cream are more functional than the pixie dust used by many companies. But without knowing the exact concentration at which they are used, it's difficult to say whether or not they are essential to the formula. If you like the way the product works for you and you can afford it, we say go for it. But if you find that it is too expensive, there are plenty of other styling products that can give you these benefits without expensive "botanicals."

Part 5: Bizarre Beauty Ingredients

Sometimes you just have to smile at the crazy concoctions that people will use on the hair and skin. From snail slime and crab shells to bird poop and bull sperm it's amazing what people are willing to try. This chapter explains which of these disgusting ingredients really work and which ones are just a waste of your time and money.

Skin care/makeup questions

Does the bird poop facial really work?

MG must know...A couple of years ago I heard a lot of buzz about the Geisha Facial that uses bird poo to improve your complexion. What's the science behind this?

We know that a lot of beauty claims are bullish*t, but this one is literally birdsh*t! Nonetheless, that hasn't stopped modern spas from adopting this ancient Japanese tradition. Shizuka New York, for example, charges you $180 for the privilege of having bird poop rubbed on your face. Supposedly, the poo brightens skin and evens out your complexion. Does it really work? Here's the scientific scoop on bird poop.

How a bird poop facial is made

First, you get some nightingales (specifically Japanese bush warblers). Why nightingales and not other birds, you ask? Because they have a short digestive tract, which allegedly allows their poop to maintain more of the chemicals that are good for your skin. Then you feed the birds a special diet of organic seeds. The seeds work their way through the birds, and what comes out the other end is called "uguisu no fun" in Japanese. Yes, that's right. The actual Japanese expression for nightingale crap that you rub all over your face includes the words "no fun." Ironic, ain't it? Next, the poop is scraped from the cages (and you thought YOU had a crappy job) and then sanitized with an ultraviolet light before being dried and ground into a fine white powder. This powder is reconstituted and used as a facial cream.

What does bird poop do for your skin?

Supposedly, bird poop contains a high concentration of urea and guanine. Urea is one of the components of the skin's Natural Moisturizing Factor (NMF for short), and it's added to a number of skin creams to improve moisturization. It really works, but you certainly don't need bird poop to get a good dose of urea! Plus, urea has to be left on the skin to provide a moisturization benefit. Leaving it for a little while and then washing it off does no good. Guanine is a naturally iridescent material that can make you look sparkly. But, again, it only works when left on your face. It doesn't have any lightening or brightening properties other than being glittery. At least one source claims that uguisu no fun contains an enzyme that lightens skin. But we could find no evidence of this at all. Most sites report that guanine is an enzyme, which it's not.

Historically, Geishas used bird poop to bleach stains from their kimonos. This makes sense, since the bird droppings could have a high pH due to ammonia, which could lighten the kinds of pigments used as fabric dyes. It won't, however, remove melanin, which is the pigment in skin that gives it its color.

THE BOTTOM LINE

Instead of wasting your money on a bird poop facial, buy a good moisturizer with urea. And if you want to get rid of acne scars or dark spots, use retinol or a skin lightener that's proven to work.

Are snail creams good for skin?

Moody muses....There is a lot of hype going on about snail creams where I live. I have friends who have used them for scar reduction/healing for acne and thought that they really did work (they got the tip from their dermatologist). I've just watched the millionth infomercial about one of these creams and am wondering if they really live up to the claims.

When we initially heard about snail extract being used in cosmetics, our BS detector kicked into overdrive. After doing a little bit of research, we're still skeptical, but at least we were able to find SOME scientific basis for using this ingredient in cosmetics.

What is snail extract?
The technical name for snail slime is "Helix Aspersa Müller Glycoconjugates." It's described as a thick fluid gathered by stimulating live snails. (We don't even WANT to know what stimulates snails.) Chemically speaking, snail slime is a complex mixture of proteoglycans, glycosaminoglycans, glycoprotein enzymes, hyaluronic acid, copper peptides, antimicrobial peptides and trace elements including copper, zinc, and iron.

The science of snail slime
There are a number of brands that claim to harness the power of snail trails. For example, there's Bioskincare, who says their product "protects, deeply moisturizes, renews and triggers the regeneration of skin damaged by acne, injuries, overstretching, photo-aging or dermatological/medical treatments." Is there any real science that supports the benefits of snail extract? Sort of.

There are certainly plenty of references in the scientific literature related to collecting snail slime. First of all, there are a number of patents related to how to gather the secretion and process it for use in cosmetics. One Chilean doctor, for example, patented a procedure for gathering the secretions by agitating snails in warm water and then filtering the mucin. Another patent, credited to a Spanish oncologist, involves stressing the snails mechanically to induce the production of their mucin. We wish we could be sure that no snails were harmed in the production of this skin cream, but based on these patents, it doesn't look good! But just because there are patents on snail slime doesn't mean it actually DOES anything. If you'll notice, the patents are related to how to collect the slime, which has nothing to do with proving it really works on your skin.

Will snail slime make wrinkles Es-car-go-away?
So does it really work? A quick Pubmed search reveals a variety of papers describing the effect of snail slime on cell cultures. In these studies, a variety of effects were seen, including the proliferation of fibroblasts, stimulation of new collagen and elastin fibers, and increased production of fibronectin proteins, to name a few. But since these effects were demonstrated on cell cultures, we have a hard time understanding how they relate to a topical cosmetic product. We did find a few other studies, though, that indicate snail extract improves skin condition by increasing the dermis' natural ability to take up and hold water. (Which makes sense, since it contains hyaluronic acid, a natural moisturizer.) And perhaps most interesting were the studies suggesting that the slime might have topical wound healing properties.

There's enough legitimate science here to make us think that snail extract may be a beneficial ingredient. However, we didn't see any data that indicates that any specific cosmetic snail cream has any special efficacy. Until we see some controlled studies of these products, we remain skeptical.

THE BOTTOM LINE
As ridiculous as this sounds at first, snail slime may be a powerful bioactive material. But translating that efficacy to a cosmetic product is another story entirely. In any given product, it's impossible to predict efficacy, because it depends on the quality of the snail extract that was used, the amount in the product, and how it's formulated and processed. Until a marketer of these products can demonstrate

they have data on their specific product, we would avoid spending a lot of money on snail creams.

Why are dead babies in my skin cream?

Helen has a hunch... My neighbor said her dermatologist gave her Neocutis, which uses PSP. Her concern was spreading dead babies on her face, and I was also interested in research regarding PSP's effect on anti-aging or wrinkle reduction. I was hoping you've already looked at this and would have a quick answer. Let me know what you think!

Thanks for a provocative question, Helen. To start with, we'll explain what PSP is.

Does PSP really come from dead babies?

PSP (or Processed Skin Proteins) is a registered trademark of Neocutis S.A. The ingredient's origins can be traced back to research conducted at University Hospital of Lausanne, Switzerland which showed that cultured fetal skin cells could speed wound healing. The cells used in the original research came from a "small biopsy of fetal skin...donated following a one-time medical termination." These original skin cells were then duplicated by culturing them in the lab and have been used to create a cosmetic version that is known as PSP. Hopefully the fact that PSP does not come directly from dead babies will help your neighbor rest a little bit easier. This is not a new issue and, not surprisingly, there has been quite a buzz in the media over using fetal-sourced material. This whole discussion will disturb some people and intrigue others, but you can click here to read more about Neocutis' responsible use of fetal skin tissue (http://thebeautybrains.com /x5mpd).

Does PSP do anything for skin?

We know from the Neocutis patent (http://thebeautybrains.com /tWDbS) that the PSP cell lysate consists of a soup of proteins and hormone-like ingredients such as "cytokines, enzymes, hormones, extracellular matrix structural proteins, neuropeptides or neuropep-tide antagonists." We also know from published research by Goldwell (http://thebeautybrains.com/qFdug), another company who works with these materials, that cytokines and human growth factors CAN improve signs of aging on skin. By about 10% to be exact. However, don't take this as conclusive evidence, since it's only a single study – there's not a ton of research in this regard.

THE BOTTOM LINE

Neocutis is not murdering babies to make their skin lotions, but that hasn't prevented them from getting a lot of bad press. And while there does to be at least some basis in scientific fact for believing that their fetal cell lystate can reduce the signs of aging, it doesn't seem to make very much of a difference. If your neighbor can spare the cash and she doesn't mind potentially being called "dead baby face," then maybe she should give it a try. Then again, she could just use a good retinol product that's been proven to work.

Is foreskin good for your face?

Kate's curious...There is a product called TNS Recovery Complex by Skin Medica that is made from (how can I say this tastefully?) a discarded piece of skin that some parents opt to have removed from their newborn baby boys before they leave the hospital. My dermatologist recommends and sells it. It has also been talked about enthusiastically on Oprah. Does this product really live up to the hype as an anti-aging, anti-wrinkle cream? It is VERY expensive!

According to the Skin Medica website, TNS contains an ingredient called NouriCel-MD, which is their tradename for a combination of Natural Growth Factors, matrix proteins, and soluble collagen. You've seen proteins and collagen before, but you may not know that Natural Growth Factors are a new category of compounds that act as chemical messengers to turn on and off a variety of cellular activities.

Natural Growth Factors for skin
Theoretically, these compounds could have anti-aging properties when used in cosmetics. However, although products like TNS do contain growth factors, it looks like this technology is still in the experimental stages. According to Dr. Farris of the American Academy of Dermatologists, "A multi-center double-blinded clinical study is currently underway to assess the anti-aging effects of human growth factors, and I expect that we'll be hearing a lot about their potential in medical applications in the coming years." Until we see study results to the contrary, we assume this product is more marketing hype than scientific breakthrough.

From foreskin?
But where did the notion that TNS contains foreskin come from? As the AAD article points out, growth factors can be extracted from plants, cultured epidermal cells, placental cells, and human foreskins. Ah ha! Since growth factors CAN be derived from foreskin (as well as other sources) and since Skin Medica uses growth factors in their TNS

product, you can see how someone could jump to the conclusion that TNS contains actual human foreskin.

In fact, according to Skin Medica, their NouriCel-MD ingredient was developed by a San Diego-based biotechnology company that patented a process for growing cell banks. So, until Skin Medica announces that their secret ingredient is really based on infant penile sheaths, our guess is that this is just another internet rumor. (Note to Skin Medica, we've already written your next ad slogan: Foreskin – For Skin!)

THE BOTTOM LINE

Upon further research, we discovered that this product contains an ingredient "engineered" from human foreskin cells. Dr. Rob Oliver, a friend of the Beauty Brains and author of the Plastic Surgery 101 blog, says it's possible that TNS contains an ingredient that is DERIVED from foreskin cells. That doesn't mean that Skin Medica is chopping up foreskins and putting them in their product.

Is charcoal good for acne?

Jolene's just asking...There's a product called Dr. Ci:Labo Basic Black Blemish Control Gel that uses charcoal to treat acne. Does it really help?

It's tough to find much information on this product, but according Dr. Ci:Labo's website: "Charcoal and gentle botanical extracts in Blemish Control Gel help to prevent the problem of oily skin by removing excess sebum." The company doesn't seem to be making any direct claims about acne, but by calling the product "Blemish Control" they're certainly implying it's good for pimples!

What causes acne?
As you probably already know, there are three different factors that cause your face to populated with pimples. Excess skin oil (sebum) production is one of the causes, but if just getting rid of oil could cure acne, all you'd have to do is wash your face. You also need to beat back the bacteria and regulate the speed at which your skin cells are sloughing off.

Can charcoal really help?
But back to Dr. Ci:Labo. Does charcoal really regulate skin oil? Highly unlikely. Charcoal doesn't have any antimicrobial properties; nor does it have the ability to regulate skin cell proliferation. The only potential mode of action is that the charcoal acts like tiny sponges to soak up oil off your face and make it magically disappear, but this is a bit hard to swallow. Besides, the oil level of your skin is self-regulating. Drying up the surface just triggers the layers beneath to produce more oil. We searched the technical literature and couldn't find ANY mention of charcoal having any beneficial skin properties.

THE BOTTOM LINE
Even if charcoal does have oil absorbing properties, that alone will not stop acne. This product may be a perfectly fine facial lotion, but unless it contains a proven anti-acne ingredient, like salicylic acid or benzoyl peroxide, it won't have any effect on zits.

Crushed bugs will make you blush

Red is the color of the blood the runs through our hearts, so it's not surprising it's always been linked to love and passion. We also see the color of passion reflected in fashion and cosmetics. Everyone has (or should have!) a sexy red lipstick or nail polish for special romantic occasions. (Revlon's Poppysilk Red Lipstick and OPI's I'm Not Really A Waitress nail polish come to mind.) These products and many others exist thanks to the miracle of modern chemistry, which has given us colorants such as FD&C Red No. 40 and D&C Red No. 33.

Natural red dye (from dead bugs)

Of course, we weren't always lucky enough to have such a rainbow of reds to choose from. Originally red dye came from a more natural, and more disgusting, source: crushed insect bodies. The cochineal insect be precise.

These bugs grow in certain varieties of cacti. They're hand picked and immersed in hot water to kill them and to dissolve waxy coating of their shells. The dead bugs are dried in the sun and then ground into a fine powder that can used as dye for fabrics, foods, and cosmetics.

THE BOTTOM LINE

Today modern chemistry can synthetically create a wide variety of red dyes, so we don't have to rely on picking bugs off cacti to make our pucker look pretty. And that's just one more reason to be thankful for cosmetic chemists!

Should I smear yogurt on my face?

Veronica asks...Can I use yogurt as a facial exfoliant because it contains an Alpha Hydroxy Acid (AHA)? I'm not sure what the concentration of AHA is in the yogurt, but the pH level is definitely under 5. So there's no need to purchase cleansers or creams containing AHA if yogurt is a natural and viable option.

We thought this was an intriguing notion and decided to look at the facts behind lactic acid in yogurt and lotions.

Is yogurt a natural exfoliant?
First the good news: the pH of yogurt is about 4.5, which IS low enough for it to be effective as an exfoliant. However, according to this food science reference, (http://www.foodsci.uoguelph.ca /dairyedu/yogurt.html) yogurt contains only about 0.9% free acid. Even if we assume that ALL the acid in yogurt is in the form of lactic acid (a common AHA), that's still a very low concentration for an active exfoliant.

How much lactic acid do skin lotions contain?
In formulated products, AHAs are used at different levels, depending on the intended effect. Regular "over the counter" exfoliant lotions contain as little as as 5 to 10% AHA. Products formulated for professional application, like chemical peels, contain much higher levels (50 to 80%). As you can see, the amount of AHA in yogurt is only a fraction of what is needed for effective exfoliation.

THE BOTTOM LINE
While it won't hurt to use yogurt on your face, it's not an effective substitute for an exfoliant with 5 to 10 times as much lactic acid.

Can I put caffeine on my skin instead of drinking coffee?

Brenda wants to know... I read about a caffeinated soap that suppos-edly gives you the same jolt as drinking coffee. Does it really work?

Brenda is referring to Shower Shock bar soap which, according to CosmeticsDesign, gives you the equivalent of 2 cups of coffee worth of caffeine every time you shower. This claim seemed a bit outrageous, so we did some digging. And guess what? Based on the published data, this is absolutely true! Imagine that – no more morning trips to Starbucks. No more messing with coffee grounds and filters! Now you can save a bundle on lattes while you lather up in the comfort of your own bathroom! Isn't that amazing???

Oh, wait a minute. There's just one catch. Bear with us here while we crunch the numbers.

Caffeine calculations

First, how much caffeine is in a cup of coffee? It's about 100 milli-grams. So for two cups, you're looking at swallowing 200 mg. Can Shower Shock match that? Let's see.

We have to establish that caffeine really does penetrate through skin into your blood. And indeed it does, according to PubMed. In fact, the diffusion rate for caffeine through human skin is 2.2 x 10-6 grams per centimeter squared of skin, per hour.

Okay, so now we know how much caffeine can penetrate 1 square centimeter of skin per hour. And since we know that the average human body has approximately 40,000 square centimeters of skin (look it up if you don't believe us!), we can calculate how much caffeine can penetrate your entire body. According to our ciphering, that means your skin can absorb about 100 mg of caffeine in about an hour. So that means you'd have to stand in the shower for 2 HOURS before you'd get the equivalent of 2 cups of coffee in your system. That trip to Starbucks doesn't seem like that bad of a deal now, does it?

THE BOTTOM LINE

Of course, we made some assumptions in this calculation, and if the fine folks who make Shower Shock would care to share their data, we'd gladly reconsider our findings. But without some kind of data to the contrary, this sounds like Marketing hype to the Beauty Brains. (And the same goes for other skin care products with caffeine, like Replenex.)

Coffee: the next big skin cosmetic ingredient

There was a recent report on research published in the journal Cancer Research, demonstrating that coffee consumption could lower your chances of developing the most common form of skin cancer. The researchers from Harvard Medical School said that their data indicates that the more coffee you consume, the less likely you are to get skin cancer.

Interesting.

Even more interesting is that the scientists isolated the effect to be from the caffeine in coffee. That should mean that beverages like soda or tea would also have a similar effect (if you adjust for caffeine levels).

The researchers caution that the data does not necessarily mean you should increase your coffee intake. They also point out that there was no protective effect from the most deadly forms of skin cancer, squamous cell carcinoma and melanoma.

So, people better keep using their sunscreen!

Adding attractive ingredients
But cosmetic marketers always need good stories to help sell products. The truth is, most cosmetic products work perfectly fine, so it takes a good story to convince consumers to buy one product over someone else's. Stories like this one would make support for a good marketing story.

Here's a system for coming up with your own bizarre new cosmetic feature ingredients.

1. Read a story about an ingredient that has shown some potential for doing something positive for skin or hair.

2. Get an extract of that ingredient and put it in your formula.

3. Publicize the ingredient that is in your formula and use scientific studies to support its use.

Of course, the ingredient probably won't improve your product significantly, but it might improve your sales. And ultimately, if you are producing excellent products, you want people to buy them. Story ingredients like these (or claims ingredients as they are called) are just the push that consumers need to try your stuff.

Are laxatives good for your skin?

Patty ponders... Tyra Banks recommends Milk of Magnesia as a makeup base in order to prevent the skin from getting oily. Will it work for acne prone skin or will it only irritate or aggravate the acne?

While we don't normally put much stock in supermodel science tips, Tyra might be on to something here.

Milk of Magnesia moves you
First, for those of you who don't know, we should explain that Milk of Magnesia (or MOM) is a common over-the-counter laxative. That's right, its main purpose is to make you poop. Technically speaking, it's a solution of magnesium hydroxide and sodium hypochlorite and it works by drawing water into the intestine to help gently pass the bowel movement. (Hey, you asked!)

Lotion from laxatives?
Interestingly, there are three reason why MOM may be beneficial to skin. One, its ability to drive water absorption into the intestines could also make it capable of tightening skin and leaving a smooth surface for makeup. Second, it has some mild antibacterial properties. And third, since it's such an effective absorbent, it may dry your skin out. Based on these properties, MOM might help against acne. But even if it works, does anyone LIKE the way it feels on their face?

A quick web search shows mixed results. Some people swear by it, saying that it keeps their makeup looking better for longer. Others say they can't stand it, because it makes their skin look and feel chalky. Our guess is that it depends on your skin type and the type of makeup you wear.

(By the way, be careful when you read what other sites say about ingredients. One forum said that MOM is a cheap alternative to Smashbox Anti-shine because it uses the same ingredient. That's not exactly true; Anti-shine contains Magnesium Aluminum Silicate, which is NOT the same as Magnesium Hydroxide.)

THE BOTTOM LINE

If you're a fan of DIY cosmetics, you might want to give Tyra's tip a try. MOM is cheap, and aside from potentially drying your skin, it's unlikely to cause you any harm.

Will snake venom smooth wrinkles?

Kari queries...I've seen several high end beauty lines that charge a small fortune for face creams that contain this synthetic snake venom, revered as the new Botox, sans injections. They claim it works just as well, albeit a bit slower, since it requires multiple applications of the cream to see results. So my questions are: does this stuff really work? If so, how does one know how much is needed for the product to actually work?

We found some interesting answers in this sell sheet about Syn-Ake. (http://thebeautybrains.com/UYgAD)f

What is Syn-ake?
Syn-ake is an anti-wrinkle material based on a synthetic tripeptide that "mimics" the effects of a peptide found in the venom of the Temple Viper snake. It was created by Pentapharm Ltd, a Swiss based chemical company. Reportedly, they are the largest snake breeders and keepers in the world too.

What does Syn-ake do?
According to the company literature, Syn-ake acts in a manner similar to a peptide in snake venom. It supposedly blocks some receptor and keeps muscles relaxed. This is supposed to smooth out your wrinkles. The relaxation of muscles is also how Botox is supposed to work.

Does it really work?
In the chemical sell sheet, data is presented from two studies. The first suggests that Syn-ake can reduce muscle cell contractions in a laboratory test. That's not in people, but in a cell culture of muscle cells. The second study shows that after 28 days of using a Syn-ake laced cream, you get a shrinkage of up to 52% of wrinkle. That must mean something, right? Well, maybe not.

Problems with the Study
The data presented as proof that Syn-ake works raises a number of questions. For example,

• What was the placebo that Syn-ake was compared to?

• Where is the proof that Syn-ake penetrates to the lower layers of the dermis where it might possibly have an effect?

• How does the performance compare to Botox or any other anti-wrinkle treatment?

• How many subjects were tested?

• Who did the testing and was it blinded?

We could go on, but there's really no point. The data presented here is incomplete and not useful for drawing conclusions. A quick search of the medical literature revealed that there were no peer reviewed studies of this ingredient. With such thin data and such incredible claims, we remain skeptical.

Then you have to add in the Marketing speak that runs throughout their press materials. Notice they don't claim that Syn-ake is a peptide found in snake venom. It only says that it "mimics the effect" of a peptide found in snake venom. It also says Syn-ake "acts in a manner similar to that of Waglerin 1? (the compound in snake venom shown to block the acetylcholine receptor).

"Mimics" and "Similar to" are weasel words that cosmetic marketing companies use when they want to create the impression that two things are related, even when they aren't. You could say body wash mimics soap, but that doesn't mean they are the same thing.

THE BOTTOM LINE

There is no credible evidence that this material works as well as Botox, no matter how much you put on your wrinkles. If you want the effectiveness of Botox, save up your money for Botox. Snake venom creams just will not be as effective.

Is eating donkey skin good for your complexion?

Melody writes...[Donkey skin] is reported to have great anti-aging effects, namely increasing elasticity of the skin, improving skin tone, preventing wrinkles and even eradicating pigmented spots.

Can donkey skin really regenerate your body? And if it can, wouldn't you be making an ass out of yourself?

Donkey dermatology

The product that MV is referring to is "Donkey Skin Gelatin" and is described as consisting of donkey skin, black sesame, walnut, dried longans and rice wine. For the sake of argument, let's assume that the product really does contain gelatin (which is made of collagen that comes from the animal hides and hooves). Does eating gelatin provide any benefits for your skin?

According to a fairly recent study (http://thebeautybrains.com /q2AF2), eating gelatin may actually help prevent some of the signs of aging. In this study, researchers at the Tokyo University of Agriculture and Technology fed gelatin to mice and measured the effect of ultraviolet light on their skin. One group of mice were fed what would be the human equivalent of one large tablespoon of gelatin everyday. They found that after 6 weeks the gelatin-ingesting mice showed a 17% increase in collagen content of their skin compared to the control group (who did not receive gelatin) who had a 53% decrease in collagen content.

THE BOTTOM LINE

This is a single study on mice, but if corroborated by further research and the appropriate clinical trials, it could indicate that eating gelatin can help your skin. Whether or not you choose to get your gelatin from slabs of donkey skin or a nice bowl of Strawberry Jell-O is up to you.

Breast milk soap: the pros and cons

Here's an idea for all you cosmetic "Do-It-Yourself-ers" out there: According to Traditionalmidwife.com, you can make your own soap using breast milk.

It's hard for us to decide if this idea is appealing or appalling. It could be appealing because there is something natural and wholesome about using mother's milk. And it could be appalling because this feels kind of like a gimmick that may not necessarily be better for your skin.

The science of soap

The recipe from the website is for a type of lye soap, which is made by neutralizing oils and fatty acids with high pH sodium hydroxide. (Lye is another name for sodium hydroxide; it's also sometimes called "caustic.") Lye soaps have been used for thousand of years, and while they do the job, they can be very harsh and drying to your skin. For this reason, they've largely been replaced by modern soap bars, which are, in fact, made with synthetic detergents. These are much milder on your skin. Modern soap bars use synthetic detergents that do not strip as much natural oil from your skin and which are not as irritating to skin proteins so they leave it better moisturized. While we give the midwife a lot of creative credit for coming up with the idea, we're not sure it's better for tender baby butts or not.

Potential issues with breast milk in soap

And here are a few other concerns you should be aware of if you're planning on making soap from breast milk.

• Be aware of the bio-hazards associated with using someone else's breast milk for soap making.

• Use precautions when handling raw, unpasteurized human milk.

• You will need to pump and store your milk in the freezer until you have at least one cup or as much as 6 cups. Add a little beer to your diet, it might help production!

• The quality and texture of frozen milk may vary after it's thawed.

THE BOTTOM LINE

Breast milk is a real ingredient in soap, but that doesn't mean it's any better for your skin than the soap bars that you can buy.

Placenta for your face

Placenta, as you know, is the nourishing lining of the uterus that is expelled after birth. In some circles, it's also a popular ingredient in beauty care products. So, here are our Top 4 things you should know about placenta and cosmetics.

Where did this crazy idea come from?

Back in the 1940s, manufacturers began promoting placental products as providing hormonal benefits like stimulating tissue growth and removing wrinkles. The FDA stepped in and ruled that these were drug claims and declared the products were ineffective and therefore illegal.

Does placenta do ANYTHING for your skin?

After the FDA's ruling, placenta suppliers changed their tune and began claiming that placental raw materials are sources of protein. Proteins are film formers and can have moisturizing benefits on hair and skin. When used at appropriate levels, this is true, but placenta proteins are no better than many other proteins that are used in hair and skin care products today.

Can placenta be harmful?

You may have heard that placenta products can give you cancer. Is this true? According to the FDA, no: placenta used in cosmetics is washed and processed many times to destroy any harmful bacteria or viruses. Besides that, the cosmetic matrix (components that bind the ingredients in products) is made from a wide variety of substances, such as alcohol and preservatives, that would present a hostile environment to any viruses or bacteria the placenta might have carried.

What about vegetable plancenta?

You're probably thinking: "Wait, placenta is the tissue that nourishes a mammal fetus during gestation. Nowhere in that fetus-nourishment definition is there any mention of plants!" Vegetable Placenta must be pure crap, right? Well guess what? Botanically speaking, there IS a vegetable placenta! According to SciScoop (http://the beautybrains.com/ifX6b), it's "the thickened portion of the inner ovary wall to which a plant's ovule(s) is (are) attached." . So it's possible to have a vegan product that contains placenta.

THE BOTTOM LINE
While you don't need to be fearful about placenta in cosmetics, there's really no substantiated reason why you should seek it out either.

Are there really crab shells in my cosmetics?

Cynthia is feeling crabby...I heard a rumor that many cosmetic products use crab shells as an ingredient. This sounds a little bit ridiculous to me, but if it's true I wonder why it's so hush-hush. Is it because the cosmetic companies are worried that the animal-rights activists will find out?

Actually, Cynthia, crab shells are a legitimate ingredient in many cosmetics.

What is Chitin?

You'll never see "crab shells" listed as an ingredient. Instead you'll see some version of a chemical called "chitin." Chitin is a polysaccharide, which means it's sort of like cellulose, and it comes from the exoskeletons of crustaceans, insects and even arachnids. When you realize this stuff could come from scorpions, suddenly crab shells don't sound so bad.

History of chitin

Chitin was "discovered" in 1811 by Professor Henri Braconnott. He found it, of all places, in the cell walls of mushrooms. We're guessing that it's too expensive to get significant amounts of high-quality chitin from mushrooms, hence the use of crustacean shells. That's much more cost effective, since these shells are a byproduct of the animals we use for food (crabs as well as shrimp and lobsters).

One of the earliest applications for chitin was in preparing wound dressings, where its moisture retention properties speed the healing of burns. Today, it's found in a variety of products, including diapers, feminine napkins, and tampons. (Since these aren't cosmetics, they don't have to provide an ingredient list.) It's also an additive in many dietary supplements and, of course, it's used in cosmetics, or else we wouldn't be writing about it.

What does chitin do in cosmetics?
It has been demonstrated that the addition of certain chitin derivatives significantly improves the skin hydrating properties of facial masks. In addition, chitin is used in hairsprays to increase combability, stiffness and curl retention. It can even help stabilize emulsions by reducing oil and water separation. Look for it on the ingredient list as either chitin or "chitosan."

THE BOTTOM LINE
While it's no secret that many products may contain ingredients derived from crustaceans, we don't think it would be a particularly wise marketing move for marketers to exclaim "Hey, I've got crabs!" Maybe that's why the animal rights groups haven't made much of a fuss about this ingredient. Somehow marine-derived ingredients seem to get a pass from the animal rights folks (with shark liver oil being a notable exception).

From the deep fat fryer to your face

According to the American Chemical Society, waste cooking oil from restaurant fryers could be the source of the next cutting edge cosmetic ingredient.

French fry face

A report by researcher Vishal Shaw in the April 9 issue of Biotechnology Progress says that cooking oil can be used to produce biosurfactants that can help regenerate damaged skin. According to Shaw et. al, United States restaurants generate about 25 billion gallons of waste cooking oil, or yellow grease, each week. Tests have shown that this grease can be transformed into chemicals known as sophorolipids that can be used in cosmetics and, interestingly, to clean fruits and vegetables.

Hmmm. Would you use a facial cleanser if you knew it was made from recycled Burger King French fry fat?

Why are there fish scales in my makeup?

Cindy's fond of fish...I read on the interwebs that nail polish is sparkly because it has ground up fish in it. Are there really fish scales in my make up?

Yes, all that's glittery and good comes from fish scales, a slice of mermaid tail, and a dash of powdered unicorn corn. Nah, we're just kidding. It really is fish scales. Sort of.

Guanine is made from fish scales
The ingredient in question is "guanine", which is indeed made from fish scales. It's related to "guano", as in bird poo, which is used to make Geisha facials. But we digress...

You'll find this ichthyotic ingredient used in makeup, bath products, cleansers, perfumes, conditioners, lipsticks, nail polishes, and so on. For legal purposes, the FDA considers guanine to be a color additive, since it imparts a sparkly, white color to cosmetics. It can also reduce the transparency of powdered products, so it's useful in makeup to cover zits and other blemishes.

Is fish safe for face?
Other than the mild gross out factor, there's nothing dangerous or toxic about putting fish scales in cosmetics. And, according to the EWG's Skin Deep Data base, guanine is "not suspected to be an environmental toxin." That's a good thing, because if it was, we'd have to EXTERMINATE ALL FISH. (Sheesh.)

As with other naturally derived ingredients, the ingredient name doesn't necessarily tell you where it comes from. You won't see "fish scales" listed on back of the pack, so look for one of these names instead: Guanine, C.I. 75170, Natural Pearl Essence or, our personal favorite, 6-Amino-6-Hydroxypurine. If you're freaked out by fish, you can look for these glittery alternatives instead: synthetic pearl, aluminum, and bronze particles. Titanium dioxide covered mica works pretty well too.

THE BOTTOM LINE

Fish scales are a real cosmetic ingredient used as a color additive. They're made as a byproduct of the fish that's used for other purposes.

Is tobacco good for your skin?

Penny pleads...How does cigarette smoke cause wrinkles?

The effects of cigarette smoke on skin have been well documented (http://thebeautybrains.com/jmBeF) elsewhere so we won't rehash that discussion here. But, it turns out that tobacco might actually be good for skin.

Tobacco road

CosmeticsDesign reports that Italian researchers have discovered a sugar-peptide found in wild tobacco plants that could have anti-aging properties for skin. This complex has antioxidant properties as well as the ability to promote collagen synthesis.

The researchers were focused on finding compounds that could protect crops from environmental stresses, but they discovered that the pathways they uncovered in plants had applications to animals as well. Specifically, they found that human keratinocytes treated with this sugar-peptide mix increased expression of two sirtuin proteins, which are thought to be linked to aging.

Will tobacco farmers everywhere breathe a sigh of relief for a more healthier use for their crops? Only time will tell.

Where can I find real blood scented perfume?

Kristen says...There was this big thing over an Italian perfumer who made a perfume that smelled like blood (http:// thebeautybrains.com/a9ELL), but really, if you look on the website, it says it's only "inspired" by it. There was also that rumor about Lady Gaga making a blood scented perfume, but again, "inspired" by blood, not actually smelling like blood. Seriously, this smell has a niche market, it would sell. Can't even find a blood scented perfume in goth stores.

Our professional technical opinion is... Yuck! Nonetheless, this question prompted an interesting discussion in our Forum.

One reader pointed out that blood doesn't really smell like anything to her. She said that "Lady Gaga perfume smells like most of other those headache inducing designer perfumes." Another responded that "even if it's not popular with the masses, if you sold it for goth punk and metal subcultures it would be a big hit! Blood does have a smell and taste; its coppery and metallic, a bit sweet from the glucose. Definitely has its own unique scent. If you have ever been to a butcher shop, you know. Mammal blood smells wonderful. Not trying to be creepy or anything, just saying it would be something I would really want to buy."

THE BOTTOM LINE
We know that fragrance houses have the ability to mimic natural scents, but we're not surprised that this technology has never been applied to the coppery odor of blood. We ARE surprised that there appears to be a market for such a scent!

Hair care questions

Can ant oil really reduce hair growth?

Talia says...There is this product called Tala Ant Egg oil; sounds fishy to me, but I am wishing it to be true!

Just when we thought we'd heard it all, here comes the invasion of the ants. Tala's Ant Egg oil is one of several products that claims to use the oil recovered from crushed ant pupae to reduce hair growth. In addition, the Tala product claims to be "tested with doctors" and "completely safe with no side effects." Is this product "excell-ant" or just ant-agonizing?

What is Ant oil?

We're cosmetic chemists, not entomologists, but as far as we've been able to figure out, Ant egg oil is really furan-2-carbaldehyde, which also known as Furfural. Apparently this stuff is a "red brown liquid and it has a sour fragrant ant smell." That's surprising, considering that Furfural is used in cosmetics as a fragrance additive! Maybe that's not a problem, since Furfural can also be derived from several non-ant sources, including wheat bran.

Regardless of the source, we couldn't find ANY published data suggesting it's effective in reducing hair growth. If this product was "tested with doctors", as Tala states, then results haven't been published in any of the standard peer reviewed databases. (As always, if someone can find a legitimate study to the contrary, we'd be happy to revise this post to reflect the new data.)

Is Ant Egg Oil safe for skin?

Not only does Furfural (apparently) not reduce hair growth, but this stuff may not be that good for your skin. It's a known skin irritant (at high concentrations), and long term exposure can lead to skin allergy and increased sunburn. Even worse, there's some concern that it may have carcinogenic properties. As a fragrance additive, Furfural is typically used at levels around 0.036%. A safety study reported by the

SCCNFP (Scientific Committee On Cosmetic Products and Non-Food Products) says that "The maximum exposure stated by RIFM does not represent any significant cancer risk. However, the exposure should not be increased." Use levels in ant egg oil creams are substantially higher than this, since its the first ingredient listed in the ingredient list. In other words, there's not much to worry about if it's in your perfume at very low levels, but it's not a good idea as a main component in a skin creme.

Ant Egg Oil Ingredients
Ant Egg Oil, Aqua,Glyceryl Stearate (and) Ceteareth-20 Ceteareth-12(and) Cetearyl Alcohol(and)Cetyl Palmitate,Herbal Extract,Dicaprylyl Carbonate,Hexyldecanol &Hexyldecayl Laurate, Glyceryl monostearate,Glycerin,Prpyle Glycol,Dimethicone, Fragrance,Phenoxiethanol,1-2-dibroma-2,4-dicyanobutane and CIT/MIT, Chamaemelum arvensis

THE BOTTOM LINE
We can't find ANY research which indicates ant egg oil has an effect on hair growth, but we did find at least one report indicating that there are some potential dangers associated with using it on the skin at high concentrations. We'd stick with a product like Vaniqua, which is proven to slow the growth of facial hair on women.

Does bull semen do anything for hair?

Manny asks...I remember reading on the webs that bull semen was the new thing to make your hair healthy looking and shiny. I was wondering if that could actually work?

Semen for hair? How do you people come up with this stuff - by watching "Something About Mary?"

Bull semen chemistry

Anyway, as everyone knows, bull semen consists of a variety of lipoproteins and nucleic acids, the most predominant being glutamic acid. Given its rather...sticky...texture, bull semen will coat the hair and provide some residual shine as long as it's not washed out. However, since hair consists of dead cells, this amino acid mixture won't provide any special rejuvenating effect. And, it certainly won't work as well as an ingredient like silicone. Considering that better alternatives exist, and given the potential sourcing issues involved with obtaining semen, we'll stick with a good shine spray.

Puns that were considered, then rejected, for this article:

• We need test-icle data to know if this works...

• We just want to disseminate the facts...

This information came from "The chemical composition of bull semen with special reference to nucleic acids, free nucleotides and free amino acids" Biochem J v.73(2); Oct 1959. Yes, that's a real reference!

Does Keratin Come From Cadavers?

Ariel says...I bet the keratin (in cosmetics) comes from cadavers.

That's an intriguing notion, in a weird "Walking Dead" kinda way....

What is keratin?
As most of you probably know, keratin is a tough type of protein from which hair, nails, hooves, and horns are made. A number of beauty products contain keratin under the assumption that adding it back to your hair will help improve its condition. (Is that true? Only if the keratin is chemically modified to stick to hair.)

Where does keratin come from?
So where does all this protein come from? From piles of bald cadavers, as Ariel suggests? Sadly, in this case, the truth is much less interesting than fiction. There are two types of keratin sold for cosmetic use. The vast majority is "regular" keratin, which comes from wool. The second type, known as human hair keratin, comes from two places. First, it can come from "reputable sources" of hair remnants. (Think beauty salons, wig makers, etc.) It does NOT come from dead bodies! Second, it can be bioengineered by using wool to duplicate the amino acid sequence of human hair.

THE BOTTOM LINE
No humans (not even dead ones) are harmed in the production of your keratin hair care products!

Are nipple creams good for your hair?

Erin asks...I use a so-called "nipple cream" on my ends and to do a pre-wash treatment once in a while. There are two different brands: Cocos Nucifera Oil and Hydrogenated Coconut Oil. Is the Cocos Nucifera Oil more likely to penetrate into the hair than the Hydrogenated Coconut Oil? What is the difference? I prefer version one, as it has Coco on top of the list (and contains some other nice things as well), but if this doesn't penetrate into the hair, it won't be that useful; what do you think?

Whew, for a minute there we you were going to ask if nipple creams where made from...well, never mind. At first glance it sounds bizarre to use nipple cream on your hair, but when you look at the chemistry, it's really not such a bad idea. Here are the ingredient lists from both of products Alex's products (she didn't provide us with the names:)

Nipple cream #1 ingredients

Hydrogenated Coconut Oil, Lanolin, Butyrosperum Parkii Butter, Cera Alba, Simmondsia Chinensis Oil, Tocopherol

Nipple cream #2 ingredients

Lanolin, Cocos Nucifera Oil, Buxus Chinensis, Tocopherol

Coconut oil quandry

In case you didn't realize it, Cocos Nucifera Oil is coconut oil (that's just the Latin name.) And here's the scoop on the hydrogenated version: When an oil is hydrogenated, the unsaturated fats (those with double carbon bond) are converted to saturated fats. In coconut oil, about 8% of the fats are unsaturated. This increases the melting point; coconut oil melts around 24°C (76 °F), whereas Hydrogenated Coconut oil will be any where from 35 to 40°C. Given that the process of hydrogenation has only changed a small part of the coconut oil, it's unlikely the performance on the hair will be significantly different to the hydrogenated form.

THE BOTTOM LINE

Based on the ingredient lists, these formulas appear to be quite similar. If both feel good on your hair, we recommend buying the cheapest one.

Part 6: Does Anything Really Work?

If you've gotten this far in the book you may be thinking that the entire beauty industry is a scam and that nothing really works as well it should. That's not true at all! There are plenty of truly functional cosmetic technologies - you just have to know where to look. This chapter helps you understand what's been really proven to work to take care of your hair and skin.

Skin care/makeup questions

Does long lasting lip color really last long?

BA begs to know...I love Covergirl Outlast All Day lip color for the summer--I can boat, pool, eat, and have lovely fresh looking lips! When I put on the lipstick, I can't help but think of nail polish, because you have to let it dry. (It's safe, right?) How in the heck does it work? AND how does the top coat make it shiny and petroleum jelly remove it?

Most long lasting lip colors stay in place because the colorants stain the skin. That approach is fine, but it means that those products can only offer a limited number of shades, because not every lip color acts as a stain. Covergirl Outlast is different from other long-lasting lip colors, because it's a two part system consisting of a colorcoat and a topcoat. Let's take a look at each.

How Outlast lasts longer

As you can see from the ingredient lists below, the color coat contains colorants in a silicone and hydrocarbon base. The topcoat is made of sucrose polycottonseedate in a waxbase. The "magic" ingredient is the sucrose material, which is a cotton seed oil ester. It's an anti-transfer agent that helps keep the color from leaving your lips. Petroleum jelly is needed to remove the waxy topcoat so you can take off the color when you're ready.

Colorgirl Outlast ingredients

All-Day Colorcoat: Isododecane, Triethylsiloxysilicate, Dimethicone, Mica, Disteardimonium Hectorite, Propylene Carbonate, Propylparaben, Simmondsia Chinensis (Jojoba) Seed Oil, Camellia Sinensis Leaf Extract, Tocopherol Acetate, Flavor, (+/- CI 15850, CI 15985, CI 19140, CI 42090, CI 73360, CI 75470, CI 77491, CI 77492, CI 77499, CI 77891)

Moisturizing Topcoat: Sucrose Polycottonseedate, Ozokerite, Cera Alba, Tocopheryl Acetate, Tocopherol, Propylparaben,

Propyl Gallate, Acetyl Glucosamine, Cocos Nucifera (Coconut Oil), Aloe Barbadensis Leaf Extract, Theobroma Cacao (Cocoa) Seed Butter, Butyrospermium Parkii (Shea Butter), Sodium Saccharin, Aroma.

THE BOTTOM LINE

Outlast does contain technology that's different from other lip colors. It's more of a hassle because you have an extra application step and it's harder to remove the color, but if all day color is what you're looking for, you should give it a try.

Will Visine help reduce skin redness?

Nelly says...I read on some other beauty website that a few drops of redness-reducing eyedrops can reduce redness and irritation from shaving. Any truth to this?

Visine (TM) is one of those products that seems to attract some wacky rumors. At one point, it was alleged that a few drops of Visine in someone's drink will induce diarrhea (not true), and it's also rumored to get rid of skin spots (it won't help with ages spots or other pigmented spots). But there does appear to be some basis for using it to temporarily reduce skin redness.

How does Visine(TM) work?

The active ingredient, tetrahydrozoline hydrochloride, reduces eye redness by constricting the superficial blood vessels in the eye. It's also used to help reduce nasal congestion. There are a couple of patents that indicate that tetrahydrozoline hydrochloride (and similar compounds) actually reduces redness (http://thebeautybrains.com/Yzyb7) from rosacea and skin erythema. (Although it appears that penetration enhancers maybe required for maximum efficacy.) We couldn't find any information on how long the effect lasts, but when used in the eye the effect lasts for 4-8 hours. Keep in mind, however, that just because the US Patent and Trademark office has approved these patents does NOT mean that the FDA has cleared the drug for this use. There is a dark side to tetrahydrozoline hydrochloride...

Watch out for side effects

There are a number of potential side effects and contraindications for this drug (http://thebeautybrains.com/cfyGy). Over exposure can cause vomiting, seizures, difficulty breathing, blurred vision and can even induce coma. Some data suggest that the drug should not be used by pregnant or nursing mothers because of potential transmission to the fetus/infant. A drop or two in the eye once in a while is safe for most people. Slathering this stuff all over your face on a frequent basis is another thing altogether!

THE BOTTOM LINE

Given the potential side effects, we'd be very careful about using this product on skin. All drugs should only be used as directed. If you have prolonged skin redness, you're better off consulting with a dermatologist to identify and treat the underlying cause.

Are probiotics good for skin?

Susan asks...I have seen some skin lotions being sold with probiotics in them. I wonder if it actually improves the skin; maybe you could just put yogurt on your face?

According to a study published in the Journal of the Society of Cosmetic Chemists, (http://thebeautybrains.com/3Chpb) certain types of probiotics are good for skin!

The benefits of probiotics

Researchers studied one probiotic in particular, Lactobacillus plantarum, a gram-positive bacteria, and found that it produces antimicrobial peptides. When used at a concentration of 5%, these peptides have antimicrobial and anti-inflammatory properties and were shown to reduce skin erythema (redness), repair the skin barrier (help lock in moisture), and reduce bad skin bacteria (that lead to acne). At a concentration of 1%, the probiotic was ineffective, so low levels won't work.

THE BOTTOM LINE

The good news is that probiotics can really work if you use enough of the right kind. The bad news is that yogurt won't have the same effect, because it contains Lactobacillus casei, a different kind of probiotic. If you want to get the right kind (Lactobacillus plantarum) from natural food products, you'd have to rub sauerkraut, pickles, brined olives, or sourdough on your face. We say go with the sourdough.

Here's a secret - these 14 cosmetics are really drugs

As long time readers of the Beauty Brains already know, cosmetics, by definition, can only affect the appearance of the body. If a product affects the physiology of the body then it's a drug, not a cosmetic. So which cosmetics fall into the drug category?

OTC Monographs
In the US, these kinds of products are called "Over The Counter drugs." The Food and Drug Administration issues Over The Counter (OTC) monographs that dictate which ingredients can be used in these products and what claims they can make. Check out the list below to learn which of your cosmetics are actually drugs.

• Anti-acne products

• Toothpaste & anti-cavity products

• Topical anti-fungal

• Anti-microbial products

• Antiperspirant

• Astringents

• Corn & Callus removers

• Dandruff products

• Hair growth / hair loss

• Nailbiting products

• Psoriasis

• Skin bleaching

• Sunscreen

• Topical analgesic

• Wart remover

Why is Gold Bond lotion good enough for stylists?

Renée asks... I'm a stylist, and I just started in a new salon. I noticed that everyone uses Gold Bond hand cream after shampooing clients' hair. I always thought that was kind of a crappy, low grade product. Shouldn't they be using a better hand cream?

Gold Bond is kind of the gold standard when it comes to protecting your hands from detergent over-exposure. That's because it contains 5 times the minimum amount of skin protectant that's required by law.

The best skin protectant ingredient
The OTC (Over The Counter drug) monograph requires that a formula contain 1% or greater of dimethicone to be considered a true skin protectant product. Since dimethicone is relatively expensive, many companies will skimp on how much they use. But Chattem, Inc, the makers of Gold Bond, use 5% dimethcone in this product, which is MUCH higher than the concentration used by many other creams and lotions. In addition, they include petrolatum, another outstanding moisture barrier ingredient. Together these two ingredients help lock moisture in the skin so it can heal itself.

To be honest, we're a little surprised to see that it also contains menthol, which, on one hand, can give a cooling effect, but, on the other hand, can irritate raw skin. If you like the way it feels, it must be working for you. In any case, this is an inexpensive product that really works – there's no need to spend more money on expensive brands.

Gold Bond Medicated Body Lotion ingredients
Active: Dimethicone 5% Menthol 0.15%

Inactive Ingredients: Water, Glycerin, Stearamidopropyl PG Dimonium Chloride Phosphate, Petrolatum, Aloe Vera (Aloe Barbadensis) Leaf Juice, Cetearyl Alcohol, Stearyl Alcohol, Distearyldimonium Chloride, Ceteareth 20, Propylene Glycol, Steareth 21, Steareth 2, Tocopheryl Acetate (Vitamin E), Diso-

dium EDTA, Imidazolidinyl Urea, Propylparaben, Methylpara-ben, Triethanolamine, Fragrance

THE BOTTOM LINE

When a cosmetic is OTC drug it will tell you how much active ingredients it contains. This information helps you pick the best product. In this case, a higher level of dimethicone creates a better skin barrier.

Which retinol product is right for me?

Rebecca asks... Is OTC retinol as good as prescription? Are they effective in the same way RX retinol is? What OTC retinol has the most effective % of retinol in the ingredients list?

This is a great question, because "retinol" is easily confused with "retinoic acid," a similar chemical that goes by a couple of different names. They both belong to a family of chemicals known as retinoids. Here's the scoop on how to keep them straight.

Not all retinoids are the same
Retinoic acid (also known as Retin-A, tretinoin and sometimes by brand names like Accutane) is a prescription drug used to treat acne. While it is primarily known for its anti-acne properties, dermatologists noticed that it can also even out complexion and reduce fine lines and wrinkles. This makes it one of the most valuable anti-aging ingredients. However, retinoic acid is not available in any cosmetic. It can only be purchased with a prescription from your doctor.

Retinol is NOT a prescription drug. It is the alcohol form of retinoic acid. That means it's chemically related and does have some similar skin refining properties; however, it is not nearly as effective as the acid.

Another problem with retinol is that it is not very stable and is easily oxidized. That means that exposure to oxygen, light, or even other ingredients in the same formula can render this ingredient even less effective.

How much retinol should I look for in cosmetic products?
You asked which over-the-counter product has the most retinol. Actually, a better question to ask is which cosmetic product has done the best job of stabilizing retinol in their formula. In the last few years, new technologies have been developed to allow formulators to stabilize retinol by encapsulating it with inert materials. If a product uses this kind of technology, their product will be more effective: a

product with 2% retinol that is not encapsulated may be less effective than a product with 0.5% retinol that is encapsulated.

THE BOTTOM LINE

Do your homework before spending a lot of money on a retinol containing face cream. Look for some reassurance that the product uses encapsulating technology to protect its precious ingredient.

Which is better, a Dove bar or a regular bar of soap?

Jackie asks...Does dove really hydrate the skin better than regular old soap? I love the scent and the creamy lather...so I probably won't stop using it even if it isn't any better, but I still would like to know if I am being ripped off by another advertising gimmick.

As far as we're concerned, a Dove bar (or even a Haagen-dazs bar) is never a rip off. Oh wait, you're talking about soap...

Dove is not a true soap (and that's good!)
Dove is what is called a "syndet" bar. That means it's a mix of synthetic detergent and soap. True soap (saponified fatty acids) can be very drying to skin, whereas modern surfactants, like Sodium Lauroyl Isethionate (SCI for short) are much less drying/irritating. As you can see from the list below, SCI is the primary ingredient in a Dove bar.

Dove Bar ingredients
Sodium Lauroyl Isethionate, Stearic Acid, Sodium Tallowate or Sodium Palmitate, Lauric Acid, Sodium Isethionate, Water, Sodium Stearate, Cocamidopropyl Betaine or Sodium C14-C16 Olefin Sulfonate, Sodium Cocoate or Sodium Palm Kernelate, Fragrance, Sodium Chloride, Tetrasodium EDTA, Tetrasodium Etidronate, Titanium Dioxide.

THE BOTTOM LINE
If you're comparing Dove to a "regular" soap bar, then yes, it's better for your skin.

Can peptides stop facial wrinkles?

Vicky asks...Which peptides in face creams are most effective in communicating with facial muscles to cause shortening of them and therefore firming the face?

According to at least one study, acetyhlexapeptide-8 is capable of reducing wrinkles associated with facial muscles.

How peptides work

This peptide allegedly works similarly to botulintoxin, aka Botox (™), by inhibiting what is known as the SNARE complex, which results in reduced muscle contractions. But unlike Botox (™), this peptide does not irreversibly destroy a key protein – its effect is temporary. Acetyhlexapeptide-8 is also supposedly able to relax the collagen and elastin matrix by altering calcium ion uptake.

THE BOTTOM LINE

We're skeptical, because we don't know the type and concentration of acetyhlexapeptide-8 used in any given product. Still, there seems to be at least some scientific basis for using this peptide to fight facial wrinkles.

What is Topical Botox?

Karen is curious...What is a topical Botox(tm)? Does it work the same way as injectable Botox(tm)? So far, how many "In-vivo" studies have been done to check the efficacy?

Topical Botox(tm)? Yeah, right. That's right up there with anti-wrinkle lotions that work like lasers, hair growth products, Bigfoot, and the Easter Bunny. Wait a minute...what's that? There's a peer reviewed, placebo-controlled study that says this might actually work?

Promising test results for topical Botox
A 2010 study conducted by Dermatology Research Institute, LLC, Coral Gables, Florida , sponsored by Revance Therapeutics, Inc., Newark, California, found botulinum toxin type A (also known as Botox(tm)) significantly decreased lateral canthal lines (LCLs also commonly known as crow's feet) when applied from a topical gel.

It's a small study (n=36 adults), but it certainly looks promising: the results, which were statistically significant at the 99% confidence interval, showed that 50% of the panelists had a decrease in LCLs by 2 units or more on an 10 unit scale compared to a placebo control (after 8 weeks). What does all that mean? Unlike so many studies on cosmetic products, this one was done with in vivo (on real people, not just in a test tube in the lab); it was done with a proper control (tested against a gel that did NOT contain the toxin); and the results where statistically significant (which is indicative that the results will be repeatable).

Stylist.com interviewed a dermatologist (http://thebeautybrains.com /bneqA) who commented on the study and raised concerns, such as the fact that the effect is much less than you will see from injectable Botox(tm), and that it's likely to only work on crow's feet, because it's easier for the toxin to penetrate the thin skin around the eyes.

THE BOTTOM LINE
Topical Botox(tm) is apparently more reliable than Bigfoot or the Easter Bunny, which is more than you can say for a lot of anti-aging products. It will be interesting to see if further testing leads to a commercially viable product.

When is it worthwhile to spend more on pressed powder?

Jennifer just wants to know...Are all pressed powder makeup products the same, or are some brands worth spending more money on?

While we stress the importance of looking at ingredients to understand the quality of a product, there are situations where the ingredients don't tell the full story. Sometimes HOW the ingredients are put together can be tremendously important to the quality of the finished product. You don't see this in simple mixtures, like shampoos, but you do see it on more complex products, like pressed powders. Case in point: a recent article in Cosmetics & Toiletries revealed that the quality of a powder cosmetic products depends in part on how the powders are pulverized.

Pulverizing powders
The powders used in cosmetics can form agglomerates, or clumps. These clumps prevent the powder from having a smooth application. To avoid these clumps, powders are processed to break them into tiny particles. This is commonly done using a piece of equipment called a "Hammer Mill", which basically slams metal hammers against the powder's surface to break the pieces apart. Most manufacturers use this type of equipment.

However, a more advanced process, known as "Jet Milling," can break the particles into even smaller sizes and make them more spherical. Not surprisingly, Jet Mills cost more and are not as readily available as Hammer Mills. That means if a company wants to make a higher quality powder, they either have to invest in more expensive equipment, or they have to use a contract manufacturer that owns this specialized grinder. In either case, the use of jet milling to create a softer-feeling product results in an increased price. Therefore, it's unlikely you'll see this used in bargain products.

THE BOTTOM LINE
While in many (most?) cases, it's not worth spending more on expensive products, there are some exceptions. If you value elegant

feel characteristics, you may want to spend more on your makeup to ensure you're getting a jet milled product. You can do a quick test to see if you like the feel of a powder by running your finger over its surface.

Is "Better Than False Lashes" mascara really better?

Karen asks...I recently read about a new Too-Faced product called "Better Than False Lashes." It uses a tube of mascara and a tube of nylon fibers. Has anyone tried this? It sounds interesting. Too-Faced promotes it as an alternative to false lashes, not as an alternative to your current mascara. Whatever. Are there any ingredients in these two products (the two tubes) that are different from other mascaras? Are there any ingredients that would make it an improvement on other mascaras?

We love to write about products with technology that differentiates them from other products. Better Than False Lashes is one of those.

How mascara works

Typical mascaras are wax-based, so they just provide a goopy thickening layer on top of your lashes. The activating mascara and top coat of Better Than False Lashes, like Blinc's Kiss Me mascara, is based on acrylic polymers, which are like hair styling gel ingredients. These polymers form a "shell" around each lash. (That's how Blinc mascara makes those little tubes.) The Flexistretch layer consists of nylon particles that give a textured effect. The combination of the two will give you an effect that is different from a regular wax based mascara.

One caveat - some people, especially contact lens wearers, have had problems with nylon fiber products, because pieces break off and get caught under the lens, resulting in eye irritation.

Better Than False Lashes Ingredients

Activating Mascara and Top Coat: Water/Aqua/Eau, Acrylates Copolymer, Propylene Glycol, Paraffin, Ozokerite, Phenyl Tri-methicone, Hydrogenated Vegetable Oil, Glyceryl Stearate SE, Stearic Acid, PVP, Glycol Montanate, Cera Alba/Beeswax/Cire d'abeille, Triethanolamine, Silica, Magnesium Aluminum Sili-cate, Hydrogenated Palm Acid, Stearyl Stearate, Synthetic Wax, Nylon-66, Phenoxyethanol, Methylparaben, Ethylpara-

ben, Propylparaben, Butylparaben, Isobutylparaben, Sodium Dehydroacetate, Black 2 (CI 77266).

Flexistretch Nylon Fibers: Nylon-66, Dimethicone, Paraffinum Liquidum/Mineral Oil/Huile minérale, Phenoxyethanol, Methylparaben, Ethylparaben, Butylparaben, Propylparaben, Isobutylparaben, Titanium Dioxide (CI 77891).

Can I use baby shampoo to remove make-up?

Laura would love to learn...Can I use baby shampoo to wash my face/remove make-up effectively? I have read on beauty blogs that you can basically just wash your face with baby shampoo (the tear-free ones) to remove even stubborn eye make-up...Is that true? We could save some serious money this way.

The Beauty Brains LOVE questions about saving money on beauty products!

3 types of makeup removers

There are three basic types of makeup removers. The first is the oil based type that remove makeup based on the principle that like dissolves like (i.e., oily stuff will dissolve oily stuff). These are typically mineral oil based. Then there's the "oil free" type, which work the same way but are based on silicones instead of mineral oil. And finally, there's the water based type that are weak solutions of mild surfactants (detergents). And guess what, that's exactly what a baby shampoo is! Here are a few examples to illustrate the point:

Makeup remover and baby shampoo ingredients

Lumene Sensitive Touch Gentle Eye Makeup Remover $5.99 for 3.4 fl oz ($1.76/oz)

> *Water, Disodium Cocoamphodiacetate, Polysorbate 20, Methylpropanediol, Glycerin, Sodium Chloride, Hydroxyethyl-cellulose, Polyaminopropyl Biguanide, Citric Acid, Linum Usita-tissimum (Linseed) Extract*

Maybelline Maybelline Expert Eyes 100% Oil Free Eye Make-Up Remover $4.49 for 2.3 fl oz ($1.95/oz)

> *Water, Propylene Glycol, Polysorbate 20, Boric Acid, Sodium Trideceth Sulfate, Disodium Lauroamphodiacetate, Hexylene Glycol, Isopropyl Alcohol, Phenylethyl Alcohol, Chlorhexidine Digluconate*

Walgreens Baby Shampoo $3.99 for 20 fl oz (19 cents/oz.)

Water, Cocamidopropyl Betaine, PEG-80 Sorbitan Laurate, So-dium Trideceth Sulfate, PEG-150 Distearate, Fragrance, Polyquaternium-10, Tetrasodium EDTA, Quaternium 15, Citric Acid, Yellow 10, Orange 4

THE BOTTOM LINE

The types of detergents used in these products are similar, and in some cases identical, to baby shampoo, yet the baby 'poo costs a LOT less. You might have to dilute the shampoo a little bit, but as long as you mix it up fresh each time, you should be fine.

(And here's another secret money saving tip: you can use baby wipes to remove makeup too.)

Can soap really kill germs?

Minnie must know...I often get contact dermatitis on my hands from soaps (liquid, soapbars or even the "mild" ones). I understand a good hygiene is necessary to prevent spreading of bacteria and virus, but how effective really is soap (surfactants) when it comes to killing germs in the first place? Is there an effective alternative that is not so irritating/dehydrating? In other words, what surfactant is the mildest on the market, and does it work on germs?

A quick literature review, courtesy of PubMed, should help answer your question.

Do you need soap?

According to a research paper entitled "The effect of handwashing with water or soap on bacterial contamination of hands" (http://thebeautybrains.com/2u5i6), water alone won't cut it (at least not for bacteria of fecal origin). The researchers found that not washing hands resulted in a 44% contamination rate. Washing with water alone dropped the contamination level to 23%, and washing with non-antibacterial soap showed only 8% contamination. So clearly, even regular soap is much better than rinsing with water alone.

Do you need antibacterial soap?

Okay, so you do need to use soap to control bacteria. But do you need special antibacterial soap? Another study (http://thebeautybrains.com/MzbiJ) found that that "although differences in efficacy between antimicrobial and non-antimicrobial soap were small, antimicrobial soap produced consistently statistically significantly greater reductions" (Ref. 2) When it comes to keeping your hands free from bacteria, it looks like soap is a MUST have and antibacterial soap is NICE to have.

THE BOTTOM LINE

If surfactant mildness is your concern, look for a hand soap (okay, actually, it's detergent, not soap) based on an ingredient called

"Sodium Cocoyl Isethionate (or SCI for short). This is one of (if not the) mildest surfactant on the market. We've blogged before about how it's used in the mildest body washes and shampoos. You can use hand sanitizers, but those are often alcohol based and may be drying to your skin.

Is stage makeup better than regular makeup?

Becky asks...I'm always on the lookout for a cosmetic product that is both better and cheaper than what I'm already using. Looking around on the internet, I read about color cosmetics and skin care lotions, made for stage and film, from brands like Graftobian, Ben Nye, Kryolan, Cinema Secrets, and Mehron. I'm tempted to try them. Has anyone had any experience with this kind of product? Also, are stage cosmetics made any differently from other makeup? Is there any reason why someone shouldn't wear them as everyday makeup?

Based on the ingredients used in stage makeup, it looks like the answer is "sometimes not different at all," "sometimes a little different," and "sometimes a lot different." How's that for a definitive response? Well, at the risk of over-elaborating, let's review a few examples from Mehron makeup, one of the self-proclaimed leaders in theatrical cosmetics.

Stage makeup composition
Not different

Let's look at the Velvet Finish Primer used to provide a smooth base for makeup application.

This product uses ingredients that are identical to those in Smashbox and other makeup primers. You know what else? Monistat bikini chafing gel makes a good makeup primer, because it uses the same ingredients! So, there's no benefit in buying special stage makeup primer.

A little different

What about more traditional makeup, like eyeshadow and lipstick? Here are two more Mehron examples. If you're a fan of reading ingredient lists (see below), these chemicals should be familiar. That's because they're the same basic ingredients used in every lipstick and eyeshadow. In the case of stage makeup, though, some ingredient levels are increased to improve longevity. While it's worth it for performers to ensure that eyeshadow doesn't crease, you may not like the way the product feels (or looks like up close). Unfortunately, the only way to know for sure is to try it for yourself.

A lot different

Greasepaint is a good example of a stage makeup that's extremely different than drug store products. Foundation Greasepaint contains pretty standard ingredients, but the oil phase is heavier than a traditional foundation. It's designed to deliver a heavy coating of pigment so that other colors can be applied on top of it (think "clown face"). It's also specially formulated not to crack or crease. You'd never wear anything this heavy or pigmented like that in your private life. (Okay, maybe you do, but we promise not to judge.)

Velvet Finish Primer Ingredients
> *Cyclomethicone, Dimethicone, Dimethicone Crosspolymer, Ascorbic Acid (Vitamin C), Aloe Barbadensis (Aloe Vera) Leaf Extract.*

Eye shadow Ingredients
> *Talc, Zinc Stearate, Magnesium Carbonate, Nylon-12, Octyl Palmitate, Dimethicone, Capric/Caprylic Triglyceride, Propylene Glycol, Diazolidinyl Urea, Methylparaben, Propylparaben.May Contain: Titanium Dioxide (CI 77891), Ultramarines (CI 77007), Iron Oxides (CI 77489), D&C Black #2 (CI 77266), FD&C Blue #1 Lake (CI 42090), Chromium Oxide Greens (CI 77288), FD&C Yellow #5 Lake (CI 19140), Mica.*

Lipstick Ingredients
> *Castor Oil, Pentaerythrityl Tetracaprylate/Tetracaprate, Hydrogenated Castor Oil / Sebacic Acid Copolymer, Candellila , C10-30 Cholesterol / Lanosterol Ester, Microcrystalline Wax, Ceresin , Carnauba , Aloe Barbadensis Leaf Extract, Tocopheryl Acetate (Vitamin E), Methylparaben, Propylparaben. May Contain: D&C Red 6 Lake (CI 15850), D&C Red 7 Lake (CI 15850), Mica.*

Foundation Greasepaint Ingredients

Mineral Oil, Ozokerite, Petrolatum, Lanolin, Isopropyl Lanolate, Sorbitan Sesquioleate, Fragrance. May Contain: Titanium Dioxide (CI 77891), D&C Red 7 Lake (CI 15850), D&C Red 6 Lake (CI 15850), Ultramarines (CI 77007), D&C Yellow 5 Lake (CI 19140), Chromium Oxide Green (CI 77288), Iron Oxides (CI 77489), Aluminum Powder (CI 77000), Mica (CI 77019), Talc.

THE BOTTOM LINE

Stage makeup is formulated with the same pallet of ingredients as regular cosmetics. In some cases, the formulas are exactly the same as drug store products. In other cases, they are amped up to be more crease resistant and sweat proof, to stand up to the rigors of performing. If you experiment, you might find some stage makeup that you like better than your regular brands. But stay away from greasepaint unless you want to end up looking like a clown.

Orange Juice and Alcohol – A New Skin Protector

We've generally been critical of the "beauty from within" trend in the cosmetic industry. There is little evidence that taking products like vitamins and herbal extracts will have any noticeable effect on the condition of your skin. Certainly, having a well-balanced diet can ensure you have healthy-looking skin, and if you are malnourished it's going to wreak havoc on your skin, but there is little evidence that when healthy people take supplements they can improve their skin.

But this doesn't mean what you eat can't have a significant impact on your skin.

Screwdriver for skin

Here's a study reported on in Dermatology Times (http://thebeautybrains.com/xL73K) that shows alcohol consumption can reduce the antioxidants in your skin and cause you to be more susceptible to sun burns. Interestingly, it took 8 minutes for the reduction in antioxidants to occur and the decrease lasted 70 minutes.

The effects were reduced when people drank the alcohol with orange juice. Presumably, scientists wanted to see how things were affected with the addition of a food that was rich in antioxidants. This indicates that if you are going to drink alcohol in the sun, be sure to have drinks that contain antioxidant rich juices. Of course, the study was done using 6 volunteers, so we wouldn't put too much faith in the conclusions. More work needs to be done.

This does suggest a new product idea for the "beauty within" trend. Could an alcohol manufacturer team up with a cosmetic company to produce skin safe cocktail mixers that people drink during outdoor festivities? Skin Safe Beer anyone?

How is sunblock different from sunscreen?

Misty asks...Do zinc oxide and titanium dioxide in products give sun protection the same way?

Yes, Misty, zinc oxide and titanium dioxide have the same mode of action: They are both minerals and they both physically scatter the rays of the sun to prevent sunburn.

How is sunblock different from sunscreen?
These minerals are generally referred to as sunblocks, which describes the mode of action of blocking the sun's rays. Compare that with the alternatives, which are typically referred to as "chemical sunscreens." (Note: To be accurate, ALL these ingredients are chemicals. And sun "block" versus sun "screen" is not strictly a technical term either. But this is how the market has historically referred to these ingredients, so we'll follow that convention for now.)

Sunscreens work by absorbing UV rays and changing them into a different wavelength of light that is not harmful to skin. Because sunscreens are chemically reactive, they can cause skin irritation, especially at higher concentrations. This is why you see so many concerns raised about chemical sunscreens and photosensitivity. Oxybenzone, octyl salicylate, and octyl methoxycinnamate are examples of UV absorbers.

Pro and con
If both types of ingredients provide the same benefit, yet chemical sunscreens have potential irritation concerns, why doesn't everyone just use mineral sunblock? Until fairly recently, the reason was that sunblocks were not very aesthetically pleasing to use. Because of their large particle size, these ingredients always left a white film on the skin. (Think of the noses of the life guards at your local pool.) In the last several years, mineral sunblocks with smaller particle sizes have been developed to reduce this whitening effect. However,

concerns have also been raised that micronized titanium oxide can penetrate the skin and cause other health issues.

THE BOTTOM LINE

Sunblocks and sunscreens work differently to accomplish the same goal. Even though the products we have right now are not perfect, they're better than risking skin cancer by wearing nothing.

Rhamnose: Anti-aging miracle or marketing ploy?

Erica asks...Vichy has created a much publicized rhamnose based anti aging line, called Liftactiv. They claim rhamnose is a very important patented discovery and that it stimulates the papillary dermis, causing it to produce new skin cells, collagen, etc. Is it true or is it the usual marketing ruse?

Vichy, for those who may not be familiar with the brand, is the self-proclaimed "number 1 skincare brand in European pharmacies." Vichy is also owned by L'Oreal, so they have access to deep pockets for R&D spending.

Liftactiv day cream
According to Vichy's website, there are 13 Liftactiv products, 3 of which contain 5% Rhamnose. (see below for the day cream ingredients)

So what's the big deal about this product? Aside from the standard "reduces the appearance of wrinkles" claims, here's what Vichy says about Liftactiv:

> "Our breakthrough formula features Rhamnose, a naturally derived plant sugar extracted in its purest form. Rhamnose in a 5% concentration has been clinically proven to improve skin rejuvenation at the source, improving collagen production, elastin production and cellular turnover."

These are pretty bold claims to make and would require significant research. Is there anything to back this up?

What does Rhamnose do?
According to a study from PubMed (http://thebeautybrains.com /rE9Ut), in vitro lab tests on cell cultures (i.e., testing done in a "glass dish"), show that cell cultures treated with rhamnose and other similar compounds produced fewer aging byproducts (known as Advanced Glycation Endproducts or AGE). These results suggest that rhamnose could be an effective anti-aging agent. Of course, laborato-

ry testing alone does not demonstrate that the benefit will be seen when used on real people, but surprisingly (at least to us), there is an in vivo study that backs up the laboratory testing.

Clinical testing

According to a paper presented by L'Oreal (http://the beautybrains.com/LReej), the effectiveness of Rhamnose has been confirmed by in vivo testing. A rhamnose containing lotion and a placebo lotion were applied twice a day for 8 weeks to the internal side of forearms of female volunteers between the ages of 50 and 70. Clinical and histological measurements were taken before and after treatment, and the results showed "a significant increase of pro-collagen I expression at papillary dermis level and considerable epidermis thickening…" This looks to be a properly designed test, but since we were unable to review the entire study protocol, we're concerned that measured effects may be statistically "significant", but may not be large enough to be observable to the user. We're still skeptical, but it's refreshing to have at least some basis for believing this technology works.

THE BOTTOM LINE

We're quick to call bullsh*t if there's no evidence of a product providing a differentiated benefit. However, in the case of Vichy's Liftactiv, based on the limited information we've been able to find, it appears that rhamnose MAY provide a measureable anti-aging benefit that other products don't. Whether or not you want to gamble $50 to find out if you can tell a difference on your skin is up to you. (You may also want to keep an eye on other, less expensive, L'Oreal brands in case they decide to leverage this technology beyond Vichy.)

Will water cure my dry, flaky scalp?

Marta muses...I have a dry scalp. My hair had a lot of dry flakes from leave in conditioner applied every day for 2 weeks. I sprayed my hair with a spray bottle of water and my dry scalp was gone. Also I sprayed my hair with water and it was so soft because of build up of leave in conditioner... After I wash my hair is it possible for me use just water to get my scalp clean and my hands to remove flakes? Also, can I just leave conditioner in my hair and react it with water? It makes so much sense, because most products contain water, and just spraying water to the product reactivates it, so I can skip applying and save product and money.

It sounds like you may be barking up the wrong tree, dry scalp-wise.

Causes of dry scalp

Spraying your hair and scalp with water certainly won't get rid of dandruff flakes. Depending on what kind of leave in conditioner you're using, though, the water could be rehydrating the dried residue from the product. As a short-term solution, this is fine, since the additional water will distribute the conditioner through your hair and temporarily refresh your style. However, it's not advisable to leave product residue on your scalp for long periods of time. This could even be contributing to scalp itching, which might make your dandruff worse.

THE BOTTOM LINE

If dry scalp/dandruff really is the cause of the flaking, try one of the over-the-counter drug dandruff shampoos that contain an active ingredient like salicylic acid, zinc pyrithione, coal tar, or selenium sulfide. To save money, buy the cheapest dandruff shampoo you can find, as long as it contains one of these approved drug ingredients.

Is salicylic acid really not effective against acne?

Sally says...Today I saw my dermatologist. When I told him that for the past 10 years I have been using salicylic acid to avoid pimples, he told me that it is now known that salicylic acid does absolutely nothing to help acne. I haven't heard this before, and honestly, it seems that I get a few pimples whenever I skip a few days of using a Paula's Choice salicylic acid product. (Is it placebo effect?) Has anyone else heard about this?

This would be a shocking development, since salicylic acid has been an approved anti-acne drug for years!

What does the recent research reveal?
We did a search of PubMed literature for recent (2010-2012) peer reviewed scientific journal articles on the subject of acne and salicylic acid. Any new discoveries about this trusted ingredient no longer working would certainly be reported here. Here's what we found:

One article (entitled Management strategies for acne vulgaris http://thebeautybrains.com/8jlqA) said "Mild acne responds favorably to topical treatments such as benzoyl peroxide, salicylic acid, and a low-dose retinoid."

Another, (Salicylic Acid Peels Versus Jessner's Solution for Acne Vulgaris: A Comparative Study http://thebeautybrains.com/s1PJj) said "In terms of noninflammatory acne lesion counts, sites treated with salicylic acid showed significant improvement."

And a third (Topical antimicrobial treatment of acne vulgaris: an evidence-based review http://thebeautybrains.com/5PCQJ) looked all the way back to 2004 and reported..."Although they have not been extensively studied, alternative agents including dapsone, salicylic acid, azelaic acid, and zinc are safe and efficacious when combined with traditional therapies."

Based on this quick review, there seems to be nothing that contradicts the conventional knowledge that salicylic acid is an effective anti-acne agent.

THE BOTTOM LINE

We're not sure where your derm is getting his or her information, but until we see evidence to the contrary, we say that salicylic acid is still effective against acne.

How can I tell which wrinkle creams really work?

Angie asks...What is your go-to anti-aging/wrinkle product? I've been trying the new StriVectin-SD for about 5 weeks now and my face feels softer and looks healthier. They say it takes about 8 weeks to see full results, so I'll let you know how it goes!

To be honest, we haven't heard great things about StriVectin, but we are big fans of testing products for ourselves rather than just accepting the marketing hype.

How to test your own wrinkle cream

Case in point: Autumn Whitefield-Madrano (who runs a terrific blog called "The Beheld"(http://www.the-beheld.com) has done a "split-face" experiment using Neutrogena Rapid Wrinkle Repair. While this kind of study doesn't take the place of a controlled clinical study, it does demonstrate the kind of critical thinking that the Beauty Brains champion. So, Autumn has graciously agreed to share her experimental results with our readers. Enjoy! (You can view Autumn's pictures on the Beauty Brains blog. http://thebeautybrains.com/KaaBS.)

Wrinkle Cream Assessment (by Autumn Whitefield-Madrano)

At age 34, I'm only just now tiptoeing into the world of anti-aging creams. My inborn skepticism has always led me to believe that most creams are snake oil—but when I started seeing fine lines creep up on my face, even snake oil viscerally seemed like it just might be worth a shot. The best way to test its efficacy—not in some company's lab, but on me? Applying anti-aging cream to half my face for a month.

The results

Well, the cream (Neutrogena Rapid Wrinkle Repair, for the curious) lived up to its eponymous claim: It did rapidly "repair" my wrinkles, to a degree. I could tell a difference in the length and depth of the fine lines that crinkle up beneath my eyes when I smile, and so could 59% of people who examined close-up photos of my face. (Only 15% of people guessed flat-out wrong; the rest couldn't tell a difference.)

Visualizing with Visia
I went in for a Visia skin analysis, which confirmed what I'd detected: There were fewer wrinkles on the treated side of my face. But when the spa director at Sensitive Touch in New York looked more carefully at the other results of my Visia scan, she advised me to stop using the cream altogether. Visia showed that I had more spots and irritation on the treated side of my face. The difference between the halves of my face wasn't dramatic—about as dramatic as the "wrinkle repair"— but it begged the question: At what point is the tradeoff of mild skin damage for mild wrinkle improvement no longer worth it?

The cream's packaging clearly instructs users to discontinue use if signs of irritation or rash appear. But as anyone who's used even a mild retinol knows, skin irritation isn't some kooky, infrequent side effect, like, say, the weird dreams that accompany anti-smoking drug Chantix. We expect that irritation—when half my face started seriously flaking a week into the experiment, I took it as par for the course. But that was just the visible side effect: Had I not had a high-tech skin analysis done, I might not have realized that my skin was continually being irritated, even after it had adjusted as seen by the naked eye. (I'll admit that the peculiarities of my experiment prevent me from getting too up in arms about it: A half-face of flaky, peeling skin is even weirder-looking than a full face of the same.) Plus, the cornucopia of sunscreen agents in this particular ensures better broad-spectrum protection...but one of those agents, homosalate, is known for drying and tightening the skin.

Pros and cons
The series of tradeoffs—broad spectrum protection for heightened chance of irritation; mild retinol benefits for mild retinol damage— might be worth it for some. Frankly, I'm not sure it's worth it for me— but I'm not sure it's not worth it, either. I think my reluctance indicates that scientific proof of a treatment's efficacy isn't really what I'm after when I spend that meditative moment applying cream every night. I'm more after the idea that I'm doing something brief

but concrete to help myself age gracefully. The cream I used has a nice feel (love that dimethicone!), making me feel like every night I was indulging myself (well, half of myself) in a feminine ritual. I know that sunscreen, yoga, and getting my five-a-day are the true routes to aging gracefully—but despite its underwhelming visible effects, I just may keep this cream as a companion along the way.

Hair care questions

Does silicone really nourish hair?

Joan asks...Could you please help with these two products (Phillip Kingsley's Elasticizer and Phytodefrisant)...are they nourishing or just bunch of silicones?

First, let's be clear about what "nourish" means in the context of hair care.

Is there a difference between "nourish" and "condition"?

You can nourish garden plants by adding water and fertilizer to the soil they grow from. But hair that has already grown out from your scalp can't be nourished like that, because it's dead. All you can really do is condition it. The definition of conditioning, according to "Conditioning Agents for Hair and Skin," is as follows:

"A product can be said to have conditioning properties if it improves the quality of the surface to which it is applied, particularly if this improvement involves correction or prevention of some aspect of surface damage."

This point is often lost because the cosmetic industry uses so many synonyms for "condition." But when it comes to hair, condition, nourish, moisturize, revitalize, replenish, restore, and vitalize all basically mean the same thing.

Which ingredients provide the best conditioning?
While it's true that some conditioning agents (like coconut oil) do have the ability to penetrate hair and help strengthen from within,

the vast majority of ingredients work by coating the hair. If left on the hair, almost any kind of oil will provide some degree of conditioning, but these can also leave hair feeling greasy and weighed down. Other ingredients, like cationic conditioners and silicones, are designed to remain on the hair after rinsing, and they provide superior lubricity and shine.

Elasticizer versus Phytodefrisant

The Phillip Kingsley product is a relatively standard rinse out conditioning treatment, which is based on silicones and cationic polymers. The Phtyo product, on the other hand, doesn't contain any traditional conditioning agents. It's all plant extracts and is designed to give your hair texture during heat styling. Since it's not rinsed out, the starchy plant materials are left in the hair, where they will provide texture. There's no scientific data, however, to back up their claim that the "straightening effect is cumulative with continued use." So, if you want the most "nourishment" for your hair, Elasticizer will give you the most benefit. If you want an "all natural" styling product, then try the Phytodefrisant Botanical Hair Relaxing Balm.

THE BOTTOM LINE

In reality, silicones are just as "nourishing" as any other ingredient that you can put on your hair.

Does Joan Rivers Great Hair Day really work?

NC asks...I have a guilty pleasure - I watch the bitchy fashion show with Joan Rivers. I heard she has some kind of miracle hair product that restores hair. More beauty BS, I assume? Come on, Brains, what's the scoop?

The product in question is "Great Hair Day" by Joan Rivers. It's essentially a colored powder that "fills in" the areas where your hair is thinner. This product is a pressed powder packaged in a compact.

Does Great Hair Day really work?
We haven't tested this specific product, but we do know that the general approach of using powder to conceal thinning hair can work with the right formula. For example, we tested Toppik Hair Building fibers and found that it works surprisingly well because it contains tiny keratin fibers that sort of "flock together" with your hair fibers. The result of this fiber building action is that Toppik actually improves the appearance of hair volume.

Compare that with the Joan Rivers' formula, which is basically talc and some polymers. It's more like a foundation than a fiber-building formula. It appears to be designed to just cover up the light covered, shiny scalp that peeks through as your hair starts to thin.

Joan Rivers Great Hair Day Ingredients
> *Talc, microcrystalline cellulose, kaolin, mica, polymathy methacyrlate, boron nitride, vp/hexadecene copolymer, fragrance, isododecane, dehydracetic acid, salicylic acid, benzoic acid, phenoxyethanol, propylene carbonate, benzyl alcohol, disteardimonium rectorate, biotin oily tripeptide-1, oleanolic acid, apigenin, peg-40 hydrogentated castor oil, ppc-26 buteth-26, water, butylene glycol, benzethonium chloride, polyquaternium-7, polyquaternium-39, methicone,*

> *May contain iron oxides, titanium dioxide, chromium oxide*

Toppik Hair Building Fibers Ingredients

Keratin, Ammonium Chloride, Silica, DMDM Hydantoin, May Contain: FD&C yellow 5, D&C red 22, D&C red 33, FD&C blue 1, D&C green 5, D&C orange 4.

THE BOTTOM LINE

If you're trying to stop your scalp from showing through thin hair, then Great Hair Day may be fine for you. If you're trying to actually make it look like you have more hair, we'd recommend Toppik. Both products have to be applied daily (assuming you wash your hair) and are about equally expensive (they'll cost around $25).

Is there such thing as a humidity resistant gel?

Monica asks... I live in MD, and even in the cold it be high humidity. My hair always get poofy in a day after I apply gel. I like my hair to be shiny, have nice defined curls, and not be crunchy. I'm African American, and if I don't use a styling gel my hair will look like a Michael Jackson bush lol. I did my own research and learned that its the PVP that draws moisture, even through I use serum with dimethicone. What ingredients are effective for holding my curls in high humidity? I read that polyquaternium -4 is supposed to be good in holding hair in humidity with little build up, soft feel , and good wet and dry combing. Also polyquaternium -11 is good, but more moisturizing, and PVP/PVA is good because of the mixture of both. I was thinking about using Aussie Instant Freezing Sculpting Gel because of the Polyquaternium 4. lol help... me....

We're always surprised to see products that still use PVP, since there are so many superior ingredients to choose from.

PVP = Polyvinylpyrrolidone
You're absolutely correct about PVP. It will give a crispy feel to your style, but it absorbs moisture like crazy, so it's not a good choice when used by itself. A PVP/VA mixture is better, but still not ideal. And the Polyquaterniums are good for soft feel and combing properties, but they don't provide a very strong hold.

So which ingredient is best for providing solid hold that's moisture resistant? The best we've ever seen is VP/Dimethylaminoethylmethacrylate Copolymer, aka Gaffix™ VC-713 (kinda just rolls off your tongue, doesn't it?) This polymer provides superior holding power even at low use levels and has outstanding high humidity resistance. Just be warned that it won't give you the same kind of crunchy feel as PVP. Here are a few products formulated with this Gaffix.

THE BOTTOM LINE

Some of the best high humidity hair gels include: Pantene Pro-V Curly Hair Style Curl Shaping Hair Gel, Extra Strong Hold TRESemme Tres Gel Extra Hold, and L'Oreal Studio Line Mega Gel, Max Hold (but it contains alcohol).

What are cationics and why are they stuck to my hair?

Gerry asks..I read that cationic surfactants stick very close to the hair because of their charge, so they can't be rinsed off with water. Which shampoo do I have to use to avoid a build up? Is a build up possible at all? Can I use soap for this, too?

"Cationic" is a chemist's way of describing a surfactant that has a positive charge. Many, but not all, cationics have a chemical name that ends in an "-ium" (like Polyquaternium-7.) There are also anionic (negatively charged) and non-ionic (non-charged) surfactants.

How do cationics condition hair?

Damaged hair has a negative charge, and opposite charges attract, so cationics make good conditioners because they will stick to the damaged spots of hair. This charge interaction helps them deposit on hair during rinsing, but the attraction is not like glue, which would make them hard to remove. It's more like the static electrical stickiness a balloon has after you rub it on a sweater. The attractive force is relatively easy to overcome, which means that washing with almost any regular shampoo will remove them. If you find that your regular shampoo feels like it's leaving something behind, that's because most shampoos these days have some conditioning agents built in. In that case, use a clarifying shampoo and you should be just fine.

By the way, as a rule of thumb you should avoid using soap on hair (especially if you have hard water), because the soap can react with the mineral ions to form a residue that leaves your hair feeling raspy and looking dull.

Does mira oil really grow hair?

FMC asks...Is mira hair oil really worth a try?

Before we answer your question, we have a question of our own: What the heck is mira oil??

What is mira oil?

It turns out that this oil has been used in India for centuries. Apparently, it's a blend of several natural plant oils. While we couldn't find an exact description of its composition, this site (http://thebeautybrains.com/hj0wK) says that mira oil contains a plant extract known as eclipta alba. One of its purported abilities of mira oil is to help hair grow faster. But does it really do anything?

The magic of mira oil

Surprise! There MAY actually be something to this stuff. We found studies published on PubMed (http://thebeautybrains.com/CjEwQ) that indicate that eclipta alba extract may stimulate hair growth. Of course, that doesn't mean that the mira oil that you buy on the internet works, because the active ingredient could be in a different form, or used at much lower concentrations, than in the published studies. For example, both studies evaluated an alcohol or ether soluble portion of the extract, not the oil soluble portion that you'd expect to find in mira oil. Still, it's an intriguing possibility.

THE BOTTOM LINE

We wouldn't rush out and spend a lot of money on mira oil until we see further research, but at least there's a kernel of scientific fact behind this product's claims.

Does any hair repair technology actually work?

Michelle asks...Are there ANY hair products out there that can actually reconstruct/repair hair (as opposed to just protecting it from further damage)?

This is a great question, because one of our pet peeves is all the products that claim to repair hair but don't. When you actually look at the science behind those products, you find that they are almost always "regular" conditioners. That means they are very good at smoothing the cuticle and helping to prevent future damage, but they do nothing to truly repair hair.

Does any hair repair product really work?
There is hope, however, because of one new technology that works differently. This technology is based on a PolyElectrolyte Complex, or PEC for short. This PEC complex consists of a negatively charged ion (PVM/MA copolymer) and a positively charged ion (Polyquaternium-28.) This combination of positive and negative charges creates a single complex with the unique ability to stick to damaged hairs and to itself.

How does PEC technology repair hair?
What does all this mean? Well, instead of just coating the outside of hair like most conditioners do, the tiny PEC molecules are able to enter the split ends of hair. Because the complex can stick to the damaged hair, protein, and other complex molecules, it creates little bridges across the open ends of the splits. As your hair dries, the water evaporates from the complex, causing it to contract. The force of this contraction pulls the end of the split hairs back together again. Once the PECs are dry, they bind the split end shut.

THE BOTTOM LINE
If you want hair repair that lasts longer than one shampoo, look for brands that sell products containing PEC technology like Nexxus, Joico, and Tresemme

Heat Protection Products For Hair

Heat styling is the most popular way to straighten and shape your hair. Unfortunately, it can also be very bad for you. This article explains why high temperature styling is bad for hair and tells you which ingredients to look for to protect your hair from heat.

Why heat is bad for hair?

Heat exposure causes three types of hair damage: 1) decomposition of hair pigment (melanin) which cause changes in hair coloration; 2) damage to the fiber surface, which makes the hair feel rough and look dull, and 3) weakening of internal hair proteins, which can result in increased breakage. These effects are greatest when hair is exposed to temperatures above 130C. Blow dryers, curlers, and flat irons are all capable of inflicting significant heat damage.

How do heat protection products work?

No one knows for sure, but here are three possible theories to explain how heat protection products work:

Uniform heat distribution

Products that leave a "buffering" layer on hair can prevent direct contact between the heating appliance and the hair surface. This protective layer can help minimize local overheating effects.

Reduced heat conduction

Almost any product that makes the hair more slippery can claim heat protection, because if the flat iron or curling iron slides through the hair more quickly, there is less likelihood of damage. This effect can reduce heat conduction and therefore decrease damage.

Oxidation-prevention

At least one study, J. Cosmet. Sci., 49, 245-256 (July/August 1998),suggests that the thermal decomposition of hair protein is caused by an oxidation reaction. Since oxidation and reduction are opposite chemical reactions, a reducing chemical like sodium bisulfite or ascorbic acid may stop the damaging reaction.

How is heat protection measured?
Heat protection can be measured using a variety of experimental techniques. Three common methods are: 1) Combing analysis to measure increases or decreases in hair surface roughness, 2) Fluorescence spectroscopy to analyze the breakdown of hair protein (usually tryptophan), and 3) Texture analysis to show changes in the mechanical properties of hair tresses.

Which ingredients really work?
There are dozens (hundreds? thousands?) of products that claim to protect hair from heat damage. Do they really work? The scientific literature shows only a few chemical compounds that have been studied and shown to provide a real, measurable benefit. For best results, look for leave-in treatment products that have these ingredients in listed toward the top of the ingredient list (in the first 5 ingredients or so):

• PVP/DMAPA acrylates copolymer

• Hydrolyzed wheat protein

• Quaternium 70

(This doesn't mean these are the ONLY ingredients in the universe that really work, but these are the only ones that have published data. Strong reducing ingredients that work by the oxidation-prevention mechanism described above are not recommended, because they may cause other types of hair damage.)

THE BOTTOM LINE
Regardless of which heat protection ingredients you choose, be careful not to confuse "heat protection" with "heat activation." Activation simply means the product undergoes some kind of change when heat is applied. Typically this refers to setting agents (in technical jargon, thermoplastic resins), which melt at the temperature of blow dryers or irons, and therefore form tighter bonds with the hair.

Does purple shampoo for silver hair really reduce brassy tones?

Donna says...Ever since I've been dying my hair blonde, I've been told by many people to treat my hair with a "purple/silver" toning shampoo or conditioner every few days to help prevent my hair from getting a brassy tone to it. Supposedly, this works by 'color theory', in that the purple toner in the shampoo is able to cancel out the brassy yellow colors in the hair. An example of such a product is the AG Sterling Silver line, one that I've been using myself (although I'm still skeptical). My question is, do these types of products actually work to keep brassy colored hair at bay?

There is a good bit of science at work here, but don't get your hopes up too high. Here's why:

The cause of yellow hair
Back in the late '60s or early '70s, companies recognized the need for shampoos focused on the problems of people with gray or silver hair. Specifically, consumers complained about their silver hair developing a yellowish cast. The yellowing effect could come from protein degradation, lipid oxidation or perhaps even residue from other haircare products. And it makes sense that it would be apparent on silver hair; subtle shifts in color are more visible on such a light background (hair that doesn't have any dark pigment). Regardless of the cause, women (and men) wanted some way to stop their silver mane from looking like it had been peed upon. (We exaggerate for dramatic effect but you get the idea.)

Colors can cancel
Enter an enterprising chemist who remembered the basic physics of the color wheel. The color wheel shows that colors that are at opposite positions have wavelengths that will cancel each other out. So, if one wanted to cancel the color yellow, one would look across it on the color wheel and find violet. Then, pulling out their trusty cosmetic ingredient dictionary, this chemist would have likely found

that a dye, External Violet 2, has two very important properties: first, it produces an intense violet color, and second, it can stain surfaces like hair and skin. Being water-soluble, Ext Violet 2 is easy to incorporate into shampoos at sufficiently high levels, where it can sustain hair. When done properly, this light violet stain is enough to counteract the yellow cast of hair, thereby returning hair to its true silver shade.

What about blond hair?
Unfortunately, the effect of violet dye shampoos on blonde hair will be very subtle, if there is any effect at all. Unlike silver hair, which has a slight yellow cast that really stands out from the background, blonde hair essentially consists of ALL yellow shades. Canceling out a little bit of yellow on a very yellow background will be a barely noticeable improvement.

AG Sterling Silver Shampoo Ingredients
> *Water/Aqua/Eau, Sodium Laureth Sulfate, Ammonium Laureth Sulfate, Cocamidopropyl Betaine, Cocamide Mea, Glycol Distearate, Laureth-10, Lauryl Pyrroudone, Hydroxypropyl Methylcellulose, Cinnamidopropyltrimonium Chloride, Dimethicone PEG-8 Meadowfomate, Helianthus Annuus (Sunflower) Extract, Calendula Officinalis Flower Extract, Lavandula Angustifolia (Lavander) Extract, Trifolium Pratense (Clover) Extract, Pinus Palustris Leaf Extract, Dianthus Cariophyllus (Carnation) Flower Extract, Panthenol, Silk Amino Acids, Cocodimonium Hydroxypropyl Hydrolyzed Keratin, Hydrolyzed Wheat Protein, Hydrolyzed Wheat Starch, Sodium PCA, Tetrasodium Edta, Ethylhexyl Methoxycinnamate, Citric Acid, Parfum/Fragrance, Methylchloroisothiazolinone, Methylisothiazolinone, Ext. Violet 2 (CI 60730), Blue 1 (CI 42090), Red 33 (CI 17200).*

THE BOTTOM LINE
All this doesn't mean you can't try it. If your hair has the right shade of yellow (brassiness), the violet may make a noticeable improve-

ment. Just be careful, because depending on the hair, the violet over yellow could give the blonde hair a greenish cast. It's advisable to try the product on a part of the hair that's not too obvious until the right routine is identified. Also, these dyes will build up if used repeatedly, and depositing too much violet dye could leave your blonde locks looking like Purple Rain.

Appendix

Where to learn more about beauty science

The Beauty Brains hope that by reading our book, everyone will become a smarter consumer who makes informed decisions when purchasing beauty products. To help you even more, here are a few examples of other great resources for finding more beauty product information and advice.

AMERICAN ACADEMY OF DERMATOLOGY

(http://www.aad.org)

This site provides a wealth of free information regarding nearly every type of skin condition known. You can find advice for how to deal with acne, eczema, psoriasis and other common skin problems. It also gives great information for finding a dermatologist in your area.

THE BEAUTY BRAINS

(http://www.thebeautybrains.com)

If you liked this book you'll LOVE our blog where you can get answers to your questions about cosmetic products. You can also learn from the questions of thousands of other people in our Forum.

CELEBRITY COSMETIC SURGERY

(http://www.celebcosmeticsurgery.com)

This blog specializes in giving you the straight dope on cosmetic surgery procedures. It's written by Dr. Anthony Youn is a Board Certified Plastic Surgeon who focuses on cosmetic surgery and celebrities.

COLIN'S BEAUTY PAGES

(http://colinsbeautypages.co.uk)

A cosmetic scientist's beauty science blog where he shares his news and views on beauty products and the science behind them

CONSUMER REPORTS

(www.consumerreports.org/cro/heQlth-fittness/beauty-personQl-care)

This is the online version of the magazine. It features information about a variety of beauty and personal care products, including researched reports on sunscreens,wrinkle creams, anti-aging products and more. It provides well-researched and unbiased information.

COSMETIC INFO

(http://www.cosmeticsinfo.org)

This is a website created by the Personal Care Products Council and contains information about the safety, testing, and regulation of cosmetics and personal care products and their ingredients. There are two section on the site including pages on ingredient safety and an ingredient database. A nice, science based alternative to the Skin Deep database.

COSMETIC, TOILETRY & PERFUMERY ASSOCIATION

(http://www.ctpa.org.uk)

This is the UK version of the Personal Care Products Council

THE EUROPEAN COMMISSION ON HEALTH AND CONCERNS

(http://ec.europa.eu/consumers/cosmetics/cosing)

Provides up do date information on the EU regulatory environment as it pertains to cosmetics.

THE FACTS ABOUT

(http://TheFactsAbout.co.uk)

This website produced by the CTPA provides reliable information about the ingredients used in cosmetics. There is information about product safety, ingredients, general cosmetic information, and specific cosmetic types.

THE FOOD AND DRUG ADMINISTRATION

(http://www.fda.gov/Cosmetics/default.htm)

Here you will find all you need to know about the regulation of cosmetics in the US. Includes safety information and a review of hot topics.

FUTURE DERM

(http://www.futurederm.com)

If you're not familiar with FutureDerm.com you should be. It's another website that embraces a science-based approached to beauty (much like The Beauty Brains.) Nicki Zevola, the owner of the site, is an aspiring dermatologist who has formulated her own line of products.

PAULA BEGOUN, THE COSMETICS COP

(http://www.paulaschoice.com/)

Paula Begoun started her career as makeup artist, moved to television as a beauty reporter and finally became the Cosmetics Cop, authoring several best books about the beauty industry, such as Don't Go to the Cosmetic Counter Without Me and The Beauty Bible. Her website and books features reviews of thousands of cosmetics and personal care products. She does an excellent job of reviewing both the products and some of the science behind.

PERSONAL CARE PRODUCTS COUNCIL-COSMETICS INFORMATION

(http://www.cosmeticsinfo.org)

This website is run by the Cosmetics Industry Oversight Council, which is responsible for ensuring that cosmetics in the U.S. comply with accepted standards. It provides good scientific information, but it is not completely unbiased, since it's run by cosmetics manufacturers.

PERSONAL CARE TRUTH

(http://personalcaretruth.com/)

Just some cosmetic industry experts providing articles about controversial topics in the cosmetic industry.

QUACK WATCH

(http://quackwatch.com)

While the site is primarily dedicated to health related topics, it provides an excellent foundation for critical thinking and evaluation of the claims, demos, and Bob used to sell cosmetics and beauty products.lent foundation for critical thinking and eva uaused to sell cosmetics and beauty products. You can find a number of articles about how to protect yourself from quackery all around you.

SOCIETY OF COSMETIC CHEMISTS

(www.scconline.org/website/news/ask_the_expert.shtml)

If you want to know more about cosmetics, try the SCC's Ask the Expert page. Simply fill out the form and send in your question. It will be answered by a member of the Society of Cosmetic Chemists.

U.S. FOOD AND DRUG ADMINISTRATION

(www.cfsan.fda.gov/~dms/cos-toc.html)

Contrary to what some sources claim, the FDA does provide regulatory guide-lines for the cosmetics industry. At this website you can find information about a number of cosmetics issues, such as ingredient and product descriptions, labeling requirements, recall information and even a quiz to test how smart you are about cosmetics.

CPSIA information can be obtained at www.ICGtesting.com
Printed in the USA
LVOW01s2357090514

385159LV00018BA/1213/P